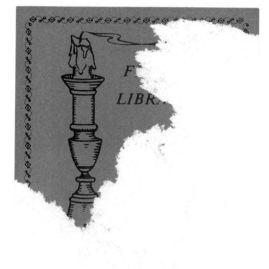

The Rape Crisis Intervention Handbook

A GUIDE FOR VICTIM CARE

The Rape Crisis Intervention Handbook

A GUIDE FOR VICTIM CARE

Edited by

SHARON L. MCCOMBIE

Director, Rape Crisis Intervention Program
Beth Israel Hospital
Boston, Massachusetts

PLENUM PRESS • NEW YORK AND LONDON

First Printing—May 1980
Second Printing—May 1983
Third Printing—August 1986

© 1980 Plenum Press, New York
A Division of Plenum Publishing Corporation
233 Spring Street, New York, N.Y. 10013

To my father
Ernest F. McCombie

Contributors

Judith H. Arons, M.S.W., A.C.S.W. ● Staff Social Worker, Obstetrics and Gynecology Service, Ambulatory Care Unit, Beth Israel Hospital; Clinical Instructor, Simmons College School of Social Work, Boston, Massachusetts

Ellen L. Bassuk, M.D. ● Assistant Professor of Psychiatry, Harvard Medical School; Director of Psychiatric Emergency Services, Beth Israel Hospital, Boston, Massachusetts

H. Jean Birnbaum, B.A. ● Consultant, Massachusetts Criminal Justice Training Council, Boston, Massachusetts

Renee S. Tankenoff Brant, M.D. ● Instructor in Psychiatry, Harvard Medical School; Director, Sexual Abuse Treatment Team, Children's Hospital Medical Center, Boston, Massachusetts

Ann Wolbert Burgess, R.N., D.N.Sc. ● Director of Nursing Research, School of Nursing, Boston University, Boston, Massachusetts; Chairperson, Rape Prevention and Control Advisory Committee, U.S. Department of Health, Education and Welfare

Janet Weeks Evans, R.N. ● Nursing Coordinator, Rape Crisis Intervention Program, Beth Israel Hospital, Boston, Massachusetts

Lynda Lytle Holmstrom, Ph.D. ● Professor and Chairperson, Department of Sociology, Boston College, Boston, Massachusetts

A. Nicholas Groth, Ph.D. ● Director, Sex Offender Program, State of Connecticut, Department of Corrections, Somers, Connecticut

Barbara Schuler Gilmore, R.N., M.S.N. ● Coordinator, Rape Service, Newton-Wellesley Hospital, Newton Lower Falls, Massachusetts

Henry Klapholz, M.D. ● Assistant Professor of Obstetrics and Gynecology, Harvard Medical School; Coordinator of Medical Education, Department of Obstetrics and Gynecology, Beth Israel Hospital, Boston, Massachusetts

Sharon L. McCombie, M.S.W., A.C.S.W. ● Founder and Director, Rape Crisis Intervention Program, Beth Israel Hospital; Clinical Instructor, Simmons College School of Social Work, Boston, Massachusetts

Catherine H. Morrison, M.S.W., A.C.S.W. ● Supervisor, Department of Social Service, Beth Israel Hospital; Clinical Instructor, Simmons College School of Social Work, Boston, Massachusetts

Peter J. Murphy, III ● Detective, Brookline Police Department, Brookline, Massachusetts

Carol C. Nadelson, M.D. ● Professor of Psychiatry, Tufts University School of Medicine; Associate-in-Chief and Director of Training and Education, Department of Psychiatry, Tufts New England Medical Center, Boston, Massachusetts

Malkah T. Notman, M.D. ● Associate Professor of Psychiatry, Harvard Medical School; Liaison Psychiatrist with Obstetrics and Gynecology, Department of Psychiatry, Beth Israel Hospital, Boston, Massachusetts

Alice E. Richmond, Esq. ● Former Assistant District Attorney, Suffolk District; former Assistant Professor, New England School of Law, Boston, Massachusetts

Daniel Silverman, M.D. ● Instructor in Psychiatry, Harvard Medical School; Director of Medical Education, Department of Psychiatry, Beth Israel Hospital, Boston, Massachusetts

Preface

This handbook is intended to be a comprehensive resource for those involved in providing crisis intervention to rape victims. The medical, legal, and counseling needs of the rape victim are presented to prepare helping professionals to offer sensitive and skillful assistance to women who have suffered sexual assault. The interdisciplinary thrust of the book reflects our conviction that health professionals, police, and prosecuting attorneys must share their expertise and coordinate their efforts in order to successfully meet the multiple needs of rape victims and their families. While an extensive literature on rape has developed in the past decade, to the best of our knowledge there is no single source for the practical treatment-oriented information sought by those who work directly with victims. The primary objective of this book is to offer just such a guide to service providers.

The book is organized into sections that deal with a specific area of the treatment of victims. Detailed guidelines are provided for the nursing, medical, counseling, police, and legal services involved in comprehensive crisis intervention. Interdisciplinary teaming and the emotional impact of rape on service providers are discussed by authors actively involved in rape crisis work. Rape laws are explained and court preparation for victim–witnesses is carefully outlined. Of particular relevance to counselors is an overview of crisis theory and a psychodynamic perspective on rape trauma. Treatment guidelines for counseling victims and their families are discussed and illustrated with case examples. We lead off with chapters that examine the cultural factors that perpetuate violence toward women and that explore common misconceptions about victims, offenders, and assaults. Although the focus of the book is on the adult woman victim, we have included a chapter on children victimized by sexual abuse. The special problems facing men who work with rape victims are addressed in the final chapter written from the point of view of the male counselor.

There are several references in the text to the appendixes of the handbook. These contain some of the educational materials we developed for the Rape Crisis Intervention Program at Beth Israel Hospital in Boston. The inclusion is not meant to indicate that these items are definitive or ideal; rather they are submitted as examples of working guidelines and fact sheets. In addition to nursing and medical protocols, we have included an example of a hospital permission form to release evidence to the police and a sample of a third-party report form for the anonymous sharing of information with the police for victims who will not report the crime to the authorities. We have included a copy of the information sheet the hospital gives to victims treated in our emergency room. There are also examples of three public education sheets that are frequently requested. The first is a questionnaire concerning myths and facts about rape that is used to encourage discussion. Another outlines the basic facts about what to do if raped, and the third lists safety precautions useful in increasing awareness about potentially risky situations.

The idea for this handbook came from our experience in training health professionals, police, and lawyers to work more effectively with rape victims. Requests for teaching and consultation evolved from the medical and counseling services we were offering to victims through the Rape Crisis Intervention Program.

Back in 1973, a small group of women mental health professionals at the Beth Israel Hospital began to organize a pilot project to provide comprehensive emergency medical and psychological assistance to women who had been raped. At that time, there was a conspicuous lack of information in the professional literature about the treatment of the adult rape victim. We found that we were largely dependent on our own resources to educate ourselves about the special needs and problems of these women. Our original interest was stimulated by the shocking frequency with which we discovered a history of a rape in the backgrounds of the women we saw in our practices. At the time of the rape, the vast majority of them had remained silent about their experience, and those who had sought assistance had usually been met with suspicions of complicity or wrongdoing. It was apparent that the original trauma of the rape was compounded by the lack of social support and services.

In the years since then, there has been an expansion in this country of services for rape victims and literature addressing the sociopolitical, epidemiological, medical, legal, and psychological issues of sexual assault. Our pilot project grew into an established Rape Crisis Intervention Program, which offers immediate and follow-up medical and counseling services to victims and their families. We have treated over 600 victims in our emergency room. The program also supplies consultation and training, provides public education to the community, and conducts ongoing clinical research on the acute and long-term impact of rape on life adjustment.

This handbook is an attempt to share the understanding we have developed from our clinical experience. There are several omissions in the book.

We do not deal with the effects of rape on homosexual women because we do not have enough direct knowledge of these victims. Also we have not addressed the needs of the male victim. While we recognize that adult males are also victims of sexual assault, the majority of those seeking services today are female. Our experience with male victims is limited, but from what we have seen, the men present the same kind of concerns and symptoms as the women we have met. They have, however, the added burden of the humiliation and fear associated with the homosexual nature of the assaults. The conspiracy of silence that kept women rape victims from our attention a decade ago still persists today for men.

Some readers may take exception to our stereotypical use of pronouns in the text. Doctors, police, and lawyers are usually referred to as "he," while nurses and counselors are designated as "she." We have followed this pattern for the sake of simplicity and readability. We do, however, fully recognize that all of these professions have both men and women among their ranks. Unfortunately, these professions still remain predominantly filled with one sex or the other. We strongly believe that men as well as women must become involved in directly helping victims as well as in changing the forces that perpetuate rape in our society. Rape and the fear and anguish it exerts will continue as long as we fail to see it as a problem that affects all of us.

This book came to be through the collective work of many people who gave generously of their energy and expertise. In addition to the work of the contributing authors, I am particularly grateful to Catherine H. Morrison for her invaluable editorial assistance and for the encouragement she provided throughout the process of developing this book. A special thanks is extended to Professor Morton D. Paley of the English Department, University of California at Berkeley, who brought his considerable editing skills and a fresh perspective to the material. The editorial contributions of Amy Schafer, Karen Shultz, Judith Arons, Andrew Gill, Donald Kalick, Maria Karagianis, and Claude Bernard were also vital to the completion of this project. I wish to thank Kate McShane for her support and secretarial assistance, and I am very grateful to Hilary Evans of Plenum for her patience and counsel throughout the preparation of the manuscript.

I am deeply appreciative of the women who used the rape crisis intervention services at the Beth Israel Hospital. It is their pain that has made this book necessary, their courage that has made it possible. I hope that what we have learned from them will contribute to helping other victims of rape.

Sharon L. McCombie

Boston

Contents

Part VII ● Appendixes

I

Myths and Realities

Rape is an act that takes place in a social milieu. Our society officially condemns those who rape, and yet our feelings toward the victim often lead us to condemn her as well. Society's reaction to rape and to its victims and perpetrators reflects deep-rooted biases and conflicting values. The myths surrounding rape must be examined, evaluated, and dispelled if we are to reduce its incidence and improve the treatment for victims. Professionals need a better understanding of both the misconceptions and the realities of rape so that effective intervention can be applied.

In this section, we begin with Catherine H. Morrison's discussion of the sociocultural aspects of rape in the context of our patriarchal society. She exposes the attitude of blaming women for rape as the logical extension of the underlying values in our social structure that have maintained women in a subordinate role to men. Examples from literature, law, psychoanalytic theory, and custom that perpetuate the inferior status of women are given to illustrate her argument that our society creates and maintains conditions that deny women full status and hence render them vulnerable to abuse. Morrison sees rape as part of a continuum of force by which persons seek to impose their will on others. Although defined as criminal, rape is only one of many kinds of oppression through which we abuse our fellow human beings. Consequently, Morrison defines rape as not just a feminist issue but a humanist concern.

A. Nicholas Groth and H. Jean Birnbaum provide us with further clarification of the mythology of rape in their report on convicted rapists. The stereotypes of the rapist as a sex-starved maniac or as a red-blooded American boy betrayed by a seductive and punitive woman are based on a view of rape as primarily motivated by sexual desire. Excerpts of conversations with offenders dramatically reveal anger and fear, rather than sexual desire, as the precipitants to the rapist's acts. Groth and Birnbaum's examination of the motives for rape leads them to conclude that rape is a sexual deviation in which sex is used to satisfy nonsexual psychic needs. They raise provocative questions regarding social policy decisions aimed at preventing rape and dealing with the offender. Their chapter is included both to assist counselors in helping victims to understand their experience and to better inform police, lawyers, policy makers, and legislators in their efforts to control rape.

Ann Wolbert Burgess and Lynda Lytle Holmstrom's chapter presents some of their findings from their pioneer study of 92 rape victims. Their report shows that for the victim, rape has little impact as a sexual act *per se;* rather, it is experienced as an act of violence and frequently as a potential murder. Excerpts from their case studies further undermine the notion that women "enjoy" rape. Where Groth and Birnbaum look at the internal dynamics of the rapists, Burgess and Holmstrom present us with a behavioral description of how assailants gain access to their victims. They also describe the various coping mechanisms and strategies used by the victims during their assaults. Their work points the way to future research to match specific survival strategies to the type of rapist and mode of attack. Police and lawyers, as well as health professionals, will find the chapter useful in increasing sophistication about women's behavioral responses to rape. Often, the victim has misgivings about her reactions during the assault. An understanding of the kind of assault and the coping model used by the victim is important in helping her to appreciate how her own behavior led to her survival.

A Cultural Perspective on Rape

Catherine H. Morrison

In the Trojan council, Paris argues against returning Helen to the Greeks:

> Sir, I propose not merely to myself
> The pleasures such a beauty brings with it;
> But I would have the soil for her fair rape
> Wiped off in honorable keeping her.
> What treason were it to the ransack'd queen,
> Disgrace to your great worths, and shame to me,
> Now to deliver her possession up
> On terms of base compulsion![1]

So goes *Troilus and Cressida,* Shakespeare's 17th-century version of Homer's *Iliad.* Written around the 10th century BC, *The Iliad* is the earliest literary work produced by Western civilization. Based as it is on the "rape" of a woman and her society's attitudes and responses to it, *The Iliad* and its various interpretations throughout history provide some interesting perspectives on the cultural context of rape.

In this context, several elementary ideas characterizing important aspects of male–female relations can be isolated. These ideas first appear in our cultural past and can be traced in variant forms to the present. Though modified and subdued, they continue to influence male–female relations and to figure predominantly in modern-day myths about rape and in personal and institutional responses to rape. These ideas are all essentially based on the notion that women, though sometimes idealized, are lesser beings than men, intrinsically inferior to them.

[1]William Shakespeare, *Troilus and Cressida,* edited by Society of Shakespearean Editors, *The Modern Readers,* Vol. 6 (New York: Bigelow, Smith and Company, 1909), pp. 53, 54.

Catherine H. Morrison ● M.S.W., A.C.S.W., Supervisor, Department of Social Service, Beth Israel Hospital; Clinical Instructor, Simmons College School of Social Work, Boston, Massachusetts.

To illustrate how these ideas relate to current rape myths and attitudes, actual quotations have been used from victims and their families, as well as from various professional and community personnel who deal with rape. These quotations were recorded by the author over a two-year period of rape counseling, in a personal journal.[2]

The first idea is that a woman, as man's inferior, finds her rightful place in society by fulfilling his destiny. She has no destiny of her own. Her role, and her pleasure, is to live out his purpose. Mythology reiterates this theme many times, for example, in Eve's creation out of Adam's rib because Adam was lonely and wanted a companion. The "rape of the Sabine women" by the founding fathers of Rome was not only forgivable but preordained and heroic on the basis of historic necessity. Even in the primary matter of procreation, the essential role was thought to be male, and women served only secondarily as receptors. In *The Eumenides* of Aeschylus, the notion is first expressed that women have no part in conception but serve simply to incubate the male's fetus. Thus, Orestes was acquitted of patricide because his mother was not a true parent. As late as the 16th century, engravings still appear of sperm drops or cells containing little, intact homunculi, curled up in the fetal position, indicating that this idea of the female's subordination in procreation still existed.

In Paris's speech quoted above, the weight of his argument as to Helen's fate rests on the importance of the preservation of male honor. Hector has entered the council saying, "She is not worth what she doth cost the holding,"[3] but later he is convinced by Paris's argument. Even though he concedes that it is morally wrong to steal and, furthermore, unwise to set such unlawful precedents among nations, he is resolved to keep Helen, to protect "our joint and several dignities."[4] Troilus then adds,

> She is a theme of honor and renown;
> A spur to valiant and magnanimous deeds,
> Whose present courage may beat down our foes,
> And fame in time to come canonize us.[5]

Modern versions of this idea appear in the tendency, at times, to take rape lightly as a crime. The assumption is that rape is in some way expectable, even "natural," as a man's superior will or his "having his way" with women is natural. This idea is carried to an extreme by some who flatly state, "There is no such thing as rape," or "Any woman who gets raped asked for it."[6] Commonly, there is the suspicion that the woman agreed to

[2]Catherine Morrison, "The Counselor's Notebook of Attitudes toward Rape," unpublished journal, 1975–1977.
[3]Shakespeare, op. cit., p. 50.
[4]Ibid., p. 55.
[5]Ibid., p. 55.
[6]Morrison, op. cit.

intercourse at the time it occurred and, for private reasons, decided later to call it rape; "It was your classic case of her changing her mind—just a little too late."[7]

Related to this same notion of women as properly furthering the male's more important life design is the idea of the heroic or "sport" rapist. This idea is currently expressed in such statements as "Young men will sow their wild oats" and "After all, what might you expect from any red-blooded young man in the back seat of a car?" or "Those boys were just out for a little fun and they found it."[8] It is expected that the modern young man, if indeed he is a man, will be honor-bound, for his dignity's sake, to find sex irresistible.

Another variant on this theme is that, deep down, a woman respects a man for overpowering her, and even enjoys it: "Women enjoy rape" or "She loved it" or, jokingly, "When you see that rape is inevitable, the best thing to do is to relax and enjoy it."[9]

The second idea that becomes focal in reviewing the cultural context of rape is also based on the idea of women as lesser beings than men. It is the idea that women actually belong to men and are their property, often, in the past, with a monetary value attached. According to this principle, women, unrelated to men, have no intrinsic value and find their value—and, again, their proper place in society—only in relation to men. Dowries and bride prices paid to fathers and husbands are one example of this idea. Susan Brownmiller, in her book *Against Our Will*,[10] did an interesting historical–legal review. She pointed out that as a result of this idea of women as male property, for thousands of years, under our culture's only extant system of laws, rape was considered not a crime against a woman but a crime against the man to whom she was financially valuable. Thus, only a virgin, who commanded a bride price, could be violated. In early Hebraic law, a man who raped an unengaged virgin could redeem himself by paying her bride price to the girl's father.

In *Troilus and Cressida,* a discussion of Helen and other chosen "wives" includes a comparison of them to goods and pieces of meat:

> Although my will distaste what it elected,
> The wife I chose? There can be no evasion
> To blench from this, and to stand firm by honor.
> We turn not back the silks upon the merchant
> When we have soiled them, nor the remainder viands

---

[7]Ibid.
[8]Ibid.
[9]Ibid.
[10]Susan Brownmiller, *Against Our Will: Men, Women and Rape* (New York: Simon & Schuster, 1975).

> We do not throw in unrespective sieve,
> Because we now are full. . . .[11]

And later:

> . . . Nature craves
> All dues be render'd to their owners: now,
> What nearer debt in all humanity
> Than wife is to the husband?[12]

This tradition of women as possessions of men, valued for their sexual "salability" or allure, continues to influence us. Since women have found their value and their place in society through their salability to a man, they have had to be careful to retain their "value." As marketable goods, they must be chaste or unsoiled, yet remain alluring enough to arouse the male market. From such a double-bind position comes the frequently expressed suspicion of women as "asking for rape" by being sexually provocative: "If she was on the street at that time of night, she must have wanted it to happen" or "Only bad women get raped" or "It doesn't happen to nice girls."[13]

The fact that rape occurred at all, in and of itself, can subtly change the attitude of people toward the victim, as well as her own attitude toward herself. It is her "fault" if it happens. She is condemned because she has failed in her social assignment to remain pure. This sense of personal failure and guilt about rape on the part of the victim has led heroines like Lucrece to suicide as the only honorable way out of having been a victim of rape. The victim's "value" has gone down, and she can seem tainted and suspect: "I used to think my daughter was a good girl, but now I don't know" or "No man can ever want me again" and "I think this will ruin me forever."[14] A husband responds, expressing both the property and the value notions, "It feels like something was taken away that belongs to me, and, now, I have it back, but used and ugly."[15]

Another popular corollary of this theme helps clarify the special suspicion with which the complaint of rape is sometimes viewed. Unlike the victim of other violent crimes such as robbery or mugging, the rape victim may have the added problem of dealing with the prejudice that "women often 'cry rape' when they are mad at their boyfriends." This idea seems to follow from the view that a woman can be "used" by a man and "dropped" instead of kept. Since she depends on him for having "the soil of her fair rape wiped off in honorable keeping," she feels "ruined" by rejection and can be driven to retaliate by accusing him of rape. Matthew Hale's famous

[11]Shakespeare, op. cit. p. 50.
[12]Ibid., p. 55.
[13]Morrison, op. cit.
[14]Ibid.
[15]Ibid.

17th-century legal commentary on the crime describes this suspicion, which can still be heard today, despite the fact that the FBI estimates rape to be the most underreported of all violent crimes, with perhaps only one in five ever coming to official attention.[16] Justice Hale said, "Rape is an accusation easily to be made and hard to be proved, and harder to be defended by the party accused, tho' never so innocent."[17]

The third idea that can be traced through our cultural development is that of women's being important to men as symbols of their power and as prizes of their prowess, thus bringing men status among their fellows, but having little to do with the relationship between the man and the woman. The more sought-after the woman, the more valuable she is to possess. Again, her value is not judged intrinsically but, in this instance, through the eyes of others, on the basis of the amount of power or status accruing to the owner from the ownership.

The Iliad opens with the famous status quarrel between Achilles and Agamemnon over the division of the spoils of war, in this case, two Trojan women. Agamemnon, forced by the gods to return his battle prize, demands immediate compensation and finally decides to confiscate Achilles' prize, "to let you know that I am more powerful than you, and to teach others not to bandy words with me and openly defy their king."[18]

Likewise, in Shakespeare's version of the Trojan council, again discussing Helen's value, Troilus exclaims,

> Is she worth keeping? Why she is a pearl,
> Whose price hath launch'd above a thousand ships,
> And turn'd crown'd kings to merchants.[19]

And in the Greek councils, Helen's worth also fluctuates, depending on the market, but always related to issues of status among men and to possession, which acclaims this status or power. For example, when the war is going badly, and the Greeks discuss leaving:

> What? Will we let Priam and the Trojans boast
> Of Argive Helen, she for whom so many Greeks
> Died before Troy, far from their native land?[20]

Again, when things go well and there is hope of negotiation:

> "For the present, let us not accept the riches of Paris;
> Nor Helen; everybody sees, even the most ignorant,

---

[16]Federal Bureau of Investigation, *Uniform Crime Reports,* 1973, p. 15.

[17]Brownmiller, op. cit., p. 369.

[18]Homer, *The Iliad,* trans. by E. V. Rieu (Harmondsworth, Middlesex: Penguin Books, 1950), p. 28.

[19]Shakespeare, op. cit., p. 55.

[20]Simone Weil, *The Iliad, or the Poem of Force,* trans. by Mary McCarthy and Dwight Macdonald, *Pendle Hill Pamphlet,* No. 91 (Wallingford, Pa., 1945), p. 23.

That Troy stands on the verge of ruin."
He spoke, and all the Achaeans acclaimed him.[21]

Modern-day variants of this idea appear in the greater social stigma attached to men for being cuckolded than to women whose husbands stray. Young men, as yet unsure of their manhood, boast of their sexual conquests to their peers. To the extent that they have been studied, group rapes provide particularly glaring examples of the use of women as symbols of male prowess. One major motive of group rape seems to be that of the participants' using women and sexuality as a way of asserting dominance in their male group.[22] In an individual rape, a victim reports of her assailant, "He said it made him feel real big doing this, powerful."[23] An inversion of the male prowess idea appears in a husband's statement: "The past few days, I've been crying a lot. All I can think about is that I'm not much of a man because it happened and I couldn't stop it."[24] Another victim, reacting to her husband after her rape, said, "I feel disgusting and dirty, but sometimes I feel he's even more disgusting because he couldn't protect me."[25]

These three basic principles of male–female relatedness, underscored by literature, have been present in our culture since its inception. The comments quoted from "The Counselor's Notebook of Attitudes toward Rape" show how modified versions of these ideas persist and help to determine some of our current responses to rape. It is also relevant to emphasize that these same attitudes show up in more ordinary, less stressful interactions than rape. They are also recognizable in common and acceptable aspects of male–female relations.

That women, as inferiors, have a service function to men is reflected in such aphorisms as "A woman's place is in the home" and "Behind every great man there is a woman." The fact that she is his sexual property, while his promiscuity is less serious, is reflected in the "double standard." Socially, a woman is encouraged to be passive and to need pampering or protection. The value aspect of the property notion is reflected in the generally accepted attitude that the female is the guardian of chastity. Her assignment is to be as seductive and marketable as possible, without actually having intercourse and spoiling the product. The old saying went "Why should he buy what he can have for free?" On the other hand, the male's prowess and dignity demand that he try as hard as possible to push the sexual issue as far as he can. The notion of women as badges of male prowess finds further expression in the general tendency of her social breed-

[21]Ibid., p. 16.
[22]Brownmiller, op. cit.
[23]Morrison, op. cit.
[24]Ibid.
[25]Ibid.

ing toward ornamental beauty and delicacy, while his is toward aggression and mastery.

Two time-honored psychiatric principles derive from the concept of women as inferior to men and in a service role to them. As modern expressions of basic cultural ideas, they deserve mention here, too. The first is the concept of penis envy, and the second is that of normal female masochism.

Sigmund Freud's theory of penis envy holds that female children spontaneously react to their first knowledge of anatomical sex differences with feelings of inferiority and loss, with the assumption that their anatomy is missing a valuable part because it lacks a penis. Little boys, on the other hand, react to this same anatomy lesson with intense fear, assuming that girls have somehow lost their penises and that this possibility exists for them as well. Freud said that the reaction of the girl is not as clear as that of the boy. "Nevertheless," he said, "we know that the female child is extremely sensitive about the lack of a sex organ equal to that of the male child. Accordingly, the girl comes to consider herself inferior to the boy, developing a condition of 'penis envy' from which may be traced a whole chain of reactions characteristic of the female."[26]

What Freud missed 100 years ago is obvious today. It is the social value of the penis that is envied and not the penis itself. Scientifically, study has never shown the male's sexual apparatus to be superior to the female's. In fact, both male and female genitalia seem to perform their respective tasks quite adequately and also to provide adequate pleasure to each. The point is that in a matriarchal society, Freud's statement could seem quite sensible read with gender reversals and the substitution of addition for lack, unequal for equal, and shame for envy. It has been the cultural disequilibrium of the two sexes and not a priori inequities that has resulted in female envy and male fear of usurpation.

Helene Deutsch formulated the theory of normal female masochism. She held that the female is anatomically passive and in some way genetically passive as well. This passivity, working together with other of her formative psychic experiences, including her usual sexual fantasies, produces an adult personality in which a degree of pleasure in suffering is not only normal but the quintessence of the healthy female specimen. Deutsch felt that this masochism is partially necessary as an accompaniment to a woman's childbearing function.[27] Here again it is curious to observe a scientist rather illogically, or unscientifically, equating such seemingly disparate elements as mental health and pleasure in suffering. Perhaps the only way pleasure in suffering could follow as mentally healthy would be when it occurred in response to a set of conditions that must be endured.

[26]Sigmund Freud, Collected Papers, Vol. 2, pp. 246–247.
[27]Helene Deutsch, The Psychology of Women: A Psychoanalytic Interpretation, Vol. 1 (New York: Grune & Stratton, 1944), pp. 276-278.

And, of course, such was the case even 100 years ago, and less, regarding the female's inferior social position.[28]

Though somewhat undermined as a result of the feminist movement, the three principles of male–female interaction reviewed above continue to stand as powerful influences in our culture. They persist still in subtly but substantially shaping our ideals of how men and women should feel, be, and relate to each other. In closely scrutinizing these three principles, there is a particular and important implication shared by each of them that needs to be addressed. In each instance, whether for the service, in the possession, or to the glory of men, women are subordinated. In each instance, women lose something of their humanity and are treated somewhat as pawns or things. With a diminution of stature and full personhood, comes inevitable manipulation and, with this, a vulnerability to misuse and to abuse.

In her essay "The Iliad, or, The Poem of Force," Simone Weil suggested that force is the central theme and the real hero of The Iliad. She defined force as that quality of interaction that turns people into things or ultimately, if exercised to its limit, human beings into corpses. Force implies the gross overriding of another's will and carries with it, however implicitly, the ultimate threat of murder. Weil argued that thus, without actually killing, force has the power to hold a human being captive, suspended, alive but unable to live, inanimate, "a thing that has a soul [which] was not made to live inside a thing; if it does so, under pressure of necessity, there is not a single element of its value to which violence is not done."[29]

Weil illustrated this point vividly by quoting from The Iliad at the moment when Hector, the most glorious of the Trojan warriors, loses his fight with Achilles. While a moment ago, he was viable, thinking, moving powerfully, now, though still living, he is reduced to a dehumanized supplicant, an object, a thing. Homer described him in this pitiable condition as

---

[28]A very interesting footnote in Deutsch's major work, The Psychology of Women, shows that she, too, was troubled by the disparity of her argument. The note answers an accusation made about her work by the "heretical" Karen Horney, who stood alone in classical analytic circles in opposition to Deutsch's theory. Horney's accusation and Deutsch's defensive answer demonstrate the ultimate conclusion of the theory of "normal female masochism." Deutsch said, "At this point, I should like to defend my previous work against a misinterpretation. K. Horney contends that I regard feminine masochism as an 'elemental power in feminine mental life' and that, according to my view, 'what woman ultimately wants in intercourse is to be raped and violated; what she wants in mental life is to be humiliated.' It is true that I consider masochism 'an elemental power in feminine life' but in my previous studies and also in this one, I have tried to show that one of woman's tasks is to govern this masochism, to steer it into the right paths, and thus to protect herself against those dangers that Horney thinks I consider woman's 'normal' lot." Cf. K. Horney, New Ways in Psychoanalysis (New York: Norton, 1938), p. 110; and Deutsch, op. cit., p. 278.

[29]Weil, op. cit., pp. 3–5.

"motionless . . . terrified, anxious to touch his knees . . . begging . . .
holding out his arms" to Achilles, who is merciless, who draws his sword
and strikes:

> Through the neck and breastbone. The two-edged sword
> Sunk home its full length. The other, face down
> Lay still, and the black blood ran out, wetting the ground.[30]

In the wonderfully uncompromising language of the poem, Achilles has
now completed and forever fixed Hector's objectification.

This moment before death is not the only time a human being can be
made to live as a thing. Weil said that Hector's fleeting agony bears the
same quality as does the whole lifetime of the slave. In both instances, a
living human being is in the power of another and, while still retaining life,
has lost the ability or right to express that life, to choose, to act freely, to
bespeak himself. For those moments, or that lifetime, he is what his master
decrees he shall be. Any misstep from ingratiation can mean sudden death.
His inner life is lost or suspended. "Force," Weil said, "in the hands of
another, exercises over the soul the same tyranny that extreme hunger does;
for it possesses, and *in perpetuo,* the power of life and death."[31]

This essay was written in the summer and fall of 1940, after the fall of
France. The author was obviously responding to that event as she focused
her attention on the dehumanizing aspects of the force of man against man
appearing in the poem. She did not deal with the obvious extension of this
force as it is applied between men and women. For our purposes, it is
important to extend her ideas in this direction, for all too often, as reflected
in the quotes from "The Counselor's Notebook," this tendency toward
"objectifying" women influences the responses of people and institutions to
the victims of rape. It even influences the responses of the rape victim
toward herself. Furthermore, the subtle ways in which women are thought
of as inferior, or are treated as "things," lie at the center of the cause of
rape.

Next to murder and slavery, kidnapping and rape stand as the ultimate
expressions of forceful objectification and dehumanization of people. What
these crimes share, in differing degrees of severity, is the gross negation of
the will of one person by another. Their relative seriousness depends on the
degree of finality or threatened finality and on the duration of time in which
this negation of will occurs. The severity of the crime corollates with the
degree to which the victim's freedom, personhood, or autonomy has been
violated.

Force, rather than sexuality, is the overriding feature of rape; and fear

---

[30]Ibid., p. 5.
[31]Ibid., p. 10.

—motionless, agonized, life-suspending fear—is the overriding response of the victims to it. This response of terror, almost universally confirmed,[32] occurs for the same reasons as does Hector's terror in facing Achilles: for whatever period the victim is detained by the assailant, his or her life is in the hands of another. His or her will is suspended, and, on threat of death, he or she is forced to serve another, to become a thing, without free will, at the disposal and at the mercy of another.

Rape is abhorrent and extreme. It is a crime in our society. Nonetheless, rape is the ultimate extension of our culture's normal tendency to regard women as inferior to men, as related to men in a useful or objective way, as servants, as possessions, or as badges of honor.

The summary of the Weil essay underscores the obvious fact that it is not only in male–female relations that force becomes a problem between people. Actually, one might view rape as the final expression of a male–female force interaction, and murder as its counterpart between men. The problem we have before us is not only a feminist one but a humanist one as well, with broad implications for injustice and exploitation of many kinds. This problem has to do with the prevalent use of force altogether in our culture.

Force or power and dehumanization or objectification exist in tandem; one cannot be without the other. If *The Iliad* is the poem of force, ours is its culture. Weil spoke to this point, commenting that in the West, the Greek idea of a penalty for the abuse of power has been lost. She noted that that idea lives on in the East as Karma, but that the West no longer even has a word to express "conceptions of limit, measure, equilibrium, which ought to determine the conduct of life."[33] Weil saw the essence of the epic and of Greek thought as contained in this concept of limit and balance, or Nemesis, as opposed to the excess and abuse of force. She saw the warriors of *The Iliad* as addicted to force, unable to extricate themselves from their own suffering, unable to end the war and go home, even when they are at moments dimly aware that the war will bring about their own ultimate destruction.

Again, speaking only of the men at battle, Weil suggested an important insight into the condition of power habituation or addiction. She said,

> Perhaps all men, by the very fact of being born, are destined to suffer violence; yet this is a truth to which circumstance shuts men's eyes. The strong are, as a matter of fact, never absolutely strong, nor are the weak absolutely weak, but neither is aware of this. They have in common a refusal to believe that they both belong to the same species: the weak see no relation between themselves and the strong, and vice versa.[34]

---

[32]Morrison, op. cit.
[33]Weil, op. cit., p. 15.
[34]Ibid., p. 13.

In this statement she seems to be pointing toward the conclusion that it is to obscure the fact of vulnerability, to attempt recompense for pain suffered, to pretend superiority over other mortals, that the warriors indulge their addiction and rush headlong into battle. Carried further, this tempting fate, this high addiction to the hope of triumph, or illusory power, is finally an effort to deny man's ultimate vulnerability. It is this that holds him in the trance of force, his attempt to deny mortality.

It is this attempt to gain the illusion of power in the face of weakness or alienation that forms the basic motivation for rape, as it does for other power plays such as war, murder, or the amassing of great empires of political or economic power. The Groth and Birnbaum chapter on the typology of rapists (Chapter 2) provides some evidence along these lines regarding convicted rapists. In *Patterns of Forcible Rape,* Menachem Amir[35] concluded that the offenders in his study, from inner-city Philadelphia, were largely young men from the lower classes and, more particularly, from the "subculture of violence." They were socially and economically deprived and depended for their status on *machismo,* which included violent and impersonal treatment of women. In the absence of other means of social or personal reward, *machismo* and violence became overvalued as perhaps the only way of expressing the Iron Rule "Do Unto Others What They Do Unto You" and of achieving in the process some temporary sense of pride or effectiveness. And rapists do not seem so different from other violent criminals. In fact, convicted rapists have usually been known to the police before for burglary (70%) and continue in criminal careers (85%), which tend to progress from burglary, to assault, to robbery, to rape, to homicide.[36] The victim who quoted her assailant above as crowing with pride and power during the rape added that afterward he cried and left her apartment. She understood his words and behavior to mean that he became dimly aware for that moment of the pathetic quality of his attempt to feel manly, masterful, or powerful.[37]

Granted, rape is a most amutual, most extreme situation. By legal definition, it is an act "against the will" of the victim. However, as an extension of other more acceptable social policies, are not women, for their part, also responsible because they suffer or support those conditions that might, in the extreme, lead to such a crime? Women also hide from ultimate vulnerabilities by finding safety in a protector's arms, just as the protector finds assurance in protection. She hitches her wagon to his star and supports him as the means for keeping herself safe.

[35]Menachem Amir, *Patterns in Forcible Rape* (Chicago: University of Chicago Press, 1971), pp. 314–331.
[36]Brownmiller, op. cit.
[37]Morrison, op. cit.

She does all this in spite of the price to herself in terms of personal freedom and fulfillment. But she does it nonetheless. Her "fulfillment" as well as her discontent rests in the fact of her subordination to her male mate. It is therefore little wonder it was finally she, via the women's movement, who began to disrupt the status quo. In the same way, it was Eve, our mythical ancestress, rather than Adam, who, as the latecomer and less enfranchised, became the dissident in the garden. It was she who proposed the eating of forbidden fruit from the tree of knowledge.

And knowledge, or wisdom, is possible. It is just not very popular in our culture. Everybody knows someone who has attained it: that special vantage point beyond self-interest where reason and passion combine to produce a world view completely objective but at the same time totally empathetic. In *The Iliad*, it is the poet himself who has attained this perspective. Weil said,

> It is in this that *The Iliad* is absolutely unique, in this bitterness that proceeds from tenderness and that spreads over the whole human race, impartial as sunlight. . . . Nothing precious is scorned, whether or not death is its destiny; everyone's unhappiness is laid bare without dissimulation or disdain; no man is set above or below the condition common to all men; whatever is destroyed is regretted. Victors and vanquished are brought equally near us; under the same head, both are seen as counterparts of the poet, and the listener as well.[38]

This condition of wisdom is true maturity. Some people do attain it, but relatively few, because generally it is not held up as a value or goal in our culture. Therefore, those who find it have more or less to stumble on it themselves.

Instead, the ideal held up for us is what Freudian psychoanalytic theory might refer to as a good Oedipal resolution. Put simply, an Oedipal resolution involves, for the male child, giving up his wish for his mother as a sexual partner, altering the aim of this wish so that he can love an available woman, and postponing its gratification until he is in reality capable of taking a sexual partner. But in this successful resolution, the basic Oedipal resolution retains Oedipal personality elements and fails to achieve the kind of maturity described above.

The basic tenets of Oedipus are: first, kingship, or a scarcity of supplies—with one mother, one father, one king or queen, and one throne or position of power; second, fierce competition for these limited supplies, people, or positions of power; and third, exploitation of others in order first to gain and then to support that scarce, hard-won power position. After all, without subjects, there can be no king. Oedipus is about kingship, not sexuality. It is about power, not love. Toward these ends, men exploit women and other men as well. The powerful or the would-be powerful

---

[38]Weil, op. cit., p. 30.

exploit the poor, the weak, the disenfranchised. Women, as well as other second-class citizens, have all too often been willing victims of the system in the hope of becoming part of the nobility, or at least courtiers in favor with a powerful prince. And in this way, people become objects, subject to manipulation and force.

The Greeks knew that this whole human dilemma was wrong. *The Iliad* is the story of epic human tragedy, of men fighting in the destructive, illusory hope of proving themselves somehow different from other men, somehow extraordinary, and therefore invulnerable, much in the way modern princes construct economic or administrative empires. But the Greeks did have an ideal higher than the power notion contained in the Oedipal situation. Juxtaposed to this human folly was always Mount Olympus, where the gods and goddesses, full of foibles, very human and very lovable, nevertheless lived rich, full lives. They betrayed their human connections by their feuds and quarrels, by their loves and special favorites among the mortals. But their own society was one in which the basic questions about mortality were solved, so that they lived together on Olympus with a great sense of community, but with each in his or her own sphere and each very respectful of the others. The idea of rape within such a community would have been absurd. While Zeus occasionally disguised himself and raped a mortal, among the gods and goddesses rape was unthinkable, and so was war. Essentially, the gods and goddesses represented the Greek notion of a greater maturity in which force could not be used between people because force had no power, because the issues of mortality and forcefulness had been resolved.

This ideal, as opposed to the one preserved by our culture in Adam and Eve's expulsion from the garden, has important consequences for the way our culture molds us. In mythological terms, the expulsion of Adam and Eve from the Garden of Eden stands for that shattering realization, that eventually comes to all men, of their own mortality. The garden represents that time in childhood characterized by a magical, symbiotic sense of fusion with the "omnipotent" parent, who, like a god, seems able to protect the child from everything. The expulsion, precipitated by eating from the Tree of Knowledge of Good and Evil, represents the loss of this innocence or naivete. It represents the awareness of nonfusion, of separation, of one's own individuality, and, with it, one's vulnerability or mortality. Adam and Eve are depicted as handling these issues by feeling rejected for some kind of sinfulness or badness of their own and by clinging to each other, half-grown and half-wise by Olympian standards, against the hardships of life until the time when they might be forgiven their sins and returned, in resurrection, to full status in their father's house, with immortality restored. They never reached an accord with death. They never faced it squarely. Instead, they only partially "separated," only partially gave up

their external ties with "omnipotent" parents, only partially accepted their
independence or full stature. They managed this by clinging to each other,
by using each other for support and for avoidance. They managed it by
essentially coming to an "Oedipal resolution." And they gave up striving
for more.

Autonomy might be defined as a stage of maturation beyond an Oedipal resolution in which self-regulation takes precedence over social adjustment or social position. Freer from external constraints, one can attain a
more perfect harmony within the self that, in turn, both permits and requires more harmony for the self within the environment. This inner (and
outer) harmony involves an acceptance of the limitations and the possibilities of the self, including an acceptance of death and other realities. Maintenance of this inner and outer harmony demands self-expression, but always
in accord with the self-expression of others. Therefore, a unity of identification with others proceeds from fuller independence and makes exploitation
of others less possible.

Full separation, ultimate mortality, and true autonomy are not dealt
with in our society. We do not see wisdom or full autonomy as values to be
attained. To the extent that we continue to stunt our growth, then power
plays and the use of force will obtain, and with them, all the destructive
implications thereof, from war, to rape, to nonconservation. Unless we
rethink our ideals and reshape our goals, we will continue not only to rape
ourselves but to kill and otherwise destroy ourselves as well, and all for the
illusory purpose of evading death. To this end, we, like the Greek warriors,
rush into battle, to our own destruction. The concept of autonomy, rather
than kingship, is the key, for force and objectification are contrary to autonomy. In this regard, the relations of men and women with each other, their
normal and their extreme or pathological relations as well, provide an important vehicle for positive change.

2

The Rapist

Motivations for Sexual Violence

A. NICHOLAS GROTH AND H. JEAN BIRNBAUM

One of the most misleading assumptions generally made with regard to men who rape is that their offenses are motivated by sexual desire. Part of the reason for this misconception is that clinicians have not studied such individuals. Rapists do not characteristically ask voluntarily for help from clinics, hospitals, or private practitioners. And those who are identified through conviction and imprisonment either do not realize that their behavior is inappropriate or symptomatic or else fear that revealing their concerns will result in their being locked up in a prison or a mental hospital. In many cases, treatment facilities are not even available to such individuals through their local community mental health agencies. Because there has been little opportunity to work with and to study a sizable number of men who rape, a body of knowledge has been slow to develop regarding this form of sexual psychopathology. In the absence of such knowledge, the exact nature of this behavior is misconstrued and misinterpreted, with the result that victimization is perpetuated rather than prevented. Without an understanding of the offender, one cannot fully appreciate what the victim experiences.

A. NICHOLAS GROTH, Ph.D. ● Director, Sex Offender Program, State of Connecticut, Department of Corrections, Somers, Connecticut.   H. JEAN BIRNBAUM, B.A. ● Consultant, Massachusetts Criminal Justice Training Council, Boston, Massachusetts.

This chapter is a condensation of some material from the book *Men Who Rape: The Psychology of the Offender* by A. Nicholas Groth with H. Jean Birnbaum, published by Plenum Publishing Corporation, 1979, and reprinted here with permission.

Rape: A Pseudosexual Act

The rapist is frequently portrayed as a lusty male who is the victim of a provocative and vindictive woman, or he is seen as a sexually frustrated man reacting under the pressure of his pent-up needs, or he is thought to be a demented sex fiend harboring insatiable and perverted desires. All these views share a common misconception: they all assume that the offender's behavior is primarily motivated by sexual desire and that rape is directed toward gratifying only this sexual need. Quite to the contrary, careful clinical study of offenders reveals that, in fact, rape serves primarily nonsexual needs. It is the sexual expression of power and anger. Forcible sexual assault is motivated more by retaliatory and compensatory motives than by sexual ones. Rape is a pseudosexual act, complex and multidetermined, but addressing issues of hostility (anger) and control (power) more than passion (sexuality). To regard rape as an expression of sexual desire is not only an inaccurate notion but an insidious assumption, for it often results in the shifting of the responsibility for the offense from the offender to the victim: if the assailant is sexually aroused and directs this arousal toward the victim, then it must be that she has deliberately or inadvertently stimulated this desire through her actions, style of dress, or some such other feature. This erroneous but popular belief that rape is the result of sexual arousal and frustration creates the foundation for a whole superstructure of related misconceptions pertaining to the offender, the offense, and the victim.

Myths about the Offender[1]

To describe the rapist as oversexed is not only an oversimplification but an inaccuracy. Rape is not an expression of sexual desire as much as it is an expression of nonsexual needs. Rape is never the result simply of sexual arousal that has no other opportunity for gratification. In fact, one-third of the offenders that we worked with were married and sexually active with their wives at the time of their assaults:

> The only way my wife and I could relate was in bed. We had good sex together, but that's all we had. We couldn't talk, we couldn't discuss things, how we felt—there was no communication.

Of those offenders who were not married (that is, single, separated, or divorced), the majority were actively involved in a variety of consenting sexual relations with other persons at the time of the offense.

[1]This section contains excerpts from A. Nicholas Groth and H. Jean Birnbaum, "Portrait of a Rapist: Is He Someone You Know?" *Pageant, 31*, No. 11 (May 1976), pp. 122–130. Copyright by Good Earth Corporation. Reprinted by permission.

Rape is always a symptom of some psychological dysfunction, either temporary and transient or chronic and repetitive. It is usually a desperate act that results from an emotionally weak and insecure individual's inability to handle the stresses and demands of his life:

> (How were you feeling at the time of the incident?) I was very depressed at the time. Empty, lonely, out-of-it feeling. I was trying like a bastard to get someone to stop me. No one listened. I wanted to kill the woman; I didn't intend to rape her. In the struggle her clothes were ripped, so I got charged with attempted rape. They showed her dress in court; it was a mess. (How did you find your victim?) How do you find a glass of beer? You go look. I was looking, but mostly I was running. (Did you try to get help?) I went to two different churches. I told everybody my history, that I had been in trouble before. I got in touch with suicide prevention and told them I didn't know whether I would act out against myself or someone else. I went to a mental hospital and got kicked out because I wasn't a resident of the state. I went to the police and was told "Fuck off." Half an hour after I left the police station, I jumped this woman. There was nothing she could have done. She tried to stop me; she tried to talk to me. She talked a lot, but I don't remember one word she said. I wanted to kill her, and when I was strangling her, I thought I heard a child cry in the next room. I stopped and apologized and left. I bought a package of razor blades and went into a theater to kill myself, and the police picked me up there.

Although rape may cut across all diagnostic categories of psychiatric disorders, the majority of such offenders are not psychotic—nor are they simply healthy and aggressive young men "sowing some wild oats." The rapist is, in fact, a person who has serious psychological difficulties that handicap him in his relationships with other people and that he discharges, when he is under stress, through sexual acting out. His most prominent defect is the absence of any close, emotionally intimate relationship with other persons, male or female. He shows little capacity for warmth, trust, compassion, or empathy, and his relationships with others are devoid of mutuality, reciprocity, and a genuine sense of sharing.

Although when he is under stress the rapist's judgment is poor, there is no problem with his intellect. He is not retarded. Why, then, does he commit such an irrational act? Out of desperation and emotional turmoil. He resorts to rape as a last desperate attempt to deal with stresses that he feels will otherwise destroy him; he often fears that he is losing control and may go insane. The consequences of his behavior, what may happen to him or to others, have no meaning at the time. Therefore, he is not deterred by such logical considerations as punishment, disgrace to his family, injury to his victim:

> I felt I had to go out and do it. I realized that sooner or later I'd get caught. I realized this would jeopardize my marriage, my job, my

freedom, yet I just had to go out and do it, as if some force deep inside me was controlling me.

Some men who ordinarily would never commit a sexual assault commit rape under very extraordinary circumstances, such as in wartime, but the likelihood of such a person's being a repetitive offender is very low. There are other men, however, who find it very difficult to meet the ordinary or usual demands of life, and the stresses that we all learn to tolerate are unendurable and overwhelming to these men. The extent to which they find most life demands frustrating, coupled with their inability to tolerate frustration and their reliance on sex as the way of overcoming their distress, makes the likelihood of their being repetitive offenders very high. Furthermore, they constitute an immediate and ongoing threat to the safety of the community. It is about them that we are most concerned and on whom this chapter is primarily focused.

Psychodynamics of Rape[2]

One of the most basic observations regarding men who rape is that not all such offenders are alike. They do not do the very same thing in the very same way or for the very same reasons. In some cases, similar acts occur for different reasons, and in other cases, different acts serve similar purposes. From our clinical experience with convicted offenders and with victims of reported sexual assault, we find that in all cases of forcible rape, three components are present: power, anger, and sexuality. The hierarchy and the interrelationships among these three factors, together with the relative intensity with which each is experienced and the variety of ways in which each is expressed, vary from one offender to another. Nevertheless, there seems to be sufficient clustering within the broad spectrum of sexual assault so that distinguishable patterns of rape can be differentiated by means of the descriptive characteristics of the assault and the dynamic characteristics of the offender.

Rape is always and foremost an aggressive act. In some offenses, the assault appears to constitute a discharge of anger; it becomes evident that the rape is the way the offender expresses and discharges a mood state of intense anger, frustration, resentment, and rage. In other offenses, the aggression seems to be reactive; that is, when the victim resists the advances of her assailant, he retaliates by striking, hitting, or hurting her in some way. Hostility appears to be quickly triggered or released, sometimes

[2]This section contains excerpts from A. Nicholas Groth, Ann Wolbert Burgess, and Lynda Lytle Holmstrom, "Rape: Power, Anger and Sexuality," *American Journal of Psychiatry*, *134*, No. 11 (November 1977), pp. 1239–1243. Copyright 1977, American Psychiatric Association. Reprinted by permission.

in a clear, consciously experienced state of anger or, in other cases, in what appears to be a panic state. In still other offenses, the aggression becomes expressed less as an anger motive and more as a means of dominating the situation—an expression of mastery and conquest. And in a fourth circumstance, the aggression itself becomes eroticized so that the offender derives pleasure from both controlling his victim and hurting her or him; that is, an intense sense of excitement and pleasure is experienced in this context whether or not actual sexual contact is made. These variations on the theme of aggression are not mutually exclusive, and in any given instance of rape, multiple meanings may be found in both the sexual and the aggressive behaviors.

In every act of rape, both aggression and sexuality are involved, and sexuality becomes the means of expressing the aggressive needs and feelings that operate in the offender and underlie his assault. Three basic patterns of rape can be distinguished: (1) the *anger rape,* in which sexuality becomes a hostile act; (2) the *power rape,* in which sexuality becomes an expression of conquest; and (3) the *sadistic rape,* in which anger and power become eroticized.

Rape is complex and multidetermined. It serves a number of psychological aims and purposes. Whatever other needs and factors operate in the commission of such an offense, however, we have found the components of anger, power, and sexuality always present and prominent. Moreover, in our experience, we find that either anger or power is the dominant component and that rape, rather than being primarily an expression of sexual desire, is, in fact, the use of sexuality to express power and anger. Rape, then, is a pseudosexual act, a pattern of sexual behavior that is concerned much more with status, hostility, control, and dominance than with sexual pleasure or sexual satisfaction. It is sexual behavior in the service of primarily nonsexual needs.

Anger Rape

In some cases of sexual assault, it is very apparent that sexuality has become a means of expressing and discharging feelings of pent-up rage. The assault is characterized by physical brutality. Far more actual force is used in the commission of the offense than would be necessary if the intent were simply to overpower the victim and achieve sexual penetration. Sex becomes the means by which the offender can degrade his victim. It is a weapon he uses to express his rage. It is his means of retaliating for what he perceives or what he has experienced as wrongs suffered at the hands of important women in his life, such as his mother or his wife. Rather than seeking sexual gratification, he is seeking to hurt, punish, degrade, and humiliate his victim, and he sees sex as a weapon to be used to this end:

Alan is a 25-year-old carpenter. Following five years of marriage and two children, his wife left him. He became depressed and began drinking and frequenting singles' bars. One evening a girlfriend with whom he had just begun an affair stood him up. He left the bar and drove to the home of an elderly lady for whom he had done some work a short time earlier. Through a ruse, he gained admittance into her house, beat her up, forced her to commit fellatio, raped her, and fled. Alan had no previous criminal record nor any history of emotional problems.

Such offenses appear to be unplanned and impulsive, and the offender, while recognizing that he was in an upset, angry, and depressed frame of mind, generally did not anticipate commiting a sexual assault. Typically, the anger rapist reports that he was not feeling sexually aroused at the time of the rape and may even have had difficulty achieving or maintaining an erection during the assault (although he had not been troubled by such impotency in his consenting relationships). His language is abusive (swearing, cursing, using obscenities, making degrading remarks), and the assault itself is of relatively short duration, sometimes over within a matter of a few minutes. The assault does discharge the offender's pent-up anger and provides temporary relief from his inner turmoil, even though he does not find the assault sexually gratifying. His anger spent, it will take time for it to build again to the critical point where he is liable to strike again, and, therefore, the sexual assaults of the anger rapist tend to be episodic. His motives are retaliation and revenge.

Power Rape

In another pattern of rape, power appears to be the dominant factor motivating the offender. In these assaults, it is not the offender's intent to harm his victim but to possess her sexually. Sexuality becomes a means of compensating for underlying feelings of inadequacy and serves to express mastery, strength, control, authority and identity. There is a desperate need on the part of the offender to reassure himself about his adequacy and competency as a man. Rape allows him to feel strong and powerful and in control of someone else. He hopes that his victim will welcome and be impressed by his sexual embrace so that he can feel that he is a sexually desirable person.

It is through sexual assault that he seeks to assert his mastery and potency and to reaffirm his identity. It is through rape that he hopes to deny deep-seated feelings of inadequacy, worthlessness, and vulnerability and to shut out disturbing doubts about his masculinity.

Warren is a single, 21-year-old sailor on furlough. He picked up a young woman hitchhiker and drove to a roadside rest area. Although she resisted his advances, he believed that "she really wanted it but didn't want me to think she was easy." He overpowered her, forced her to submit to intercourse, and afterward asked her for a date later that same evening. Warren had committed four similar offenses in the space of a week but had no previous criminal or psychiatric history.

Such offenses are preplanned although the actual assault may depend on opportunity. Adult sexuality is threatening to such an offender since it confronts him with issues of adequacy and competency, and at the time of the assault, he is usually anxious. The power rapist, too, does not find the offense sexually pleasurable because it never lives up to his fantasy, and he may experience a premature or retarded ejaculation during the assault. His language is instructional (giving orders and commands) and inquisitive (asking the victim personal questions), and the assault may be of an extended duration. Although the power rapist may claim that he was motivated by sexual desire, an examination of his offense typically reveals no effort to negotiate a consenting encounter—he then would not be in control —nor any attempts at foreplay or lovemaking. Instead his modus operandi is capture, control, and conquer. Not feeling in control of his own life, the power rapist attempts to deny his feelings of helplessness and vulnerability by having sexual control of someone else.

Sadistic Rape

In a third pattern of rape, both sexuality and aggression are fused into a single psychological experience known as *sadism*. Aggression itself is eroticized, and this offender finds the deliberate and intentional sexual abuse of his victim intensely exciting and gratifying. Such assaults usually involve bondage and torture, ritualistic behaviors, and symbolic victims (that is, the victims seem to share some common characteristic in appearance or profession). In some cases, the offender is an individual who cannot achieve sexual satisfaction unless his victim physically resists him; he becomes aroused or excited only when aggression is present, and he finds pleasure in taking a woman against her will. In extreme cases, the sadistic rapist may murder his victim and mutilate her body. In less extreme cases, he may, rather than have actual intercourse with her, use some type of object or instrument to rape her, such as a stick or a bottle:

> Eric is a 30-year-old divorced man charged with first-degree murder. His victim, a 20-year-old woman he picked up at a singles' bar, was tied to a tree, whipped, raped, sodomized, and slashed to death. Although found to be sane, Eric claimed that he was high on drugs and couldn't remember what had happened. He had a criminal record that included assault and battery, breaking and entering, nonsupport, and motor vehicle violations. At the age of 17, he had tied a 13-year-old neighbor girl to a bed and assaulted her. He beat his children and

burned his wife with cigarettes during intercourse. Shortly after his conviction, Eric committed suicide.

Rape, then, is not the aggressive expression of sexuality as much as it is the sexual expression of aggression. To this end, it may serve several motives in the psychology of the offender: rape may be experienced as a way of hurting (anger), of defiling (contempt), of controlling (mastery), of exploiting (power), and of destroying (sadism). What is gratifying to the rapist is not sexual release *per se* but the discharge of anger, the feeling of power, or the sense of excitement he derives from the offense. Rape, rather than being primarily or essentially an expression of sexual desire, is in fact the use of sex to express anger, power, domination, exploitation, and retaliation. The recognition of these various determinants in the psychology of the offender may help counselors to appreciate the full impact of the assault on the victim. Dispelling the myths and misconceptions about the offender and his offense should help to prevent the compounding of the victim's victimization.

Myths about Responses to Rape[3]

It is frequently believed that if a woman really wanted to, she could always prevent the assault. The fact is that rape occurs through intimidation with a weapon, threat of harm or injury, or brute force. Different motives operate in different offenders, and therefore, what might be successful in dissuading one type of assailant might, in fact, only encourage a different type. Physical resistance discourages one kind of rapist but excites another type. If his victim screams, one assailant will flee, but another will cut her throat.

Again, since rape is commonly thought to be aimed at satisfying a simple sexual urge, the remedies often proposed address themselves to simple sexual needs. For example, it is sometimes suggested that one way to stop rape is to legalize prostitution. The fact is that prostitution does exist, but it offers no solution because the offender is not seeking primarily sexual gratification. Prostitutes themselves are sometimes the victims of rape, since they may represent qualities the rapist finds threatening and resents in women.

Rape is sometimes attributed to the increasing availability of pornography and sexual explicitness in the public media. Although a rapist, like anyone else, might find some pornography stimulating, it is not sexual

[3]This section contains excerpts from A. Nicholas Groth and H. Jean Birnbaum, "Portrait of a Rapist: Is He Someone You Know?" *Pageant, 31,* No. 11 (May 1976), pp. 122–130. Copyright by Good Earth Corporation. Reprinted by permission.

arousal but the arousal of anger or fear that leads to rape. Pornography does not cause rape; banning it will not stop rape. In fact, some studies have shown that rapists are generally exposed to less pornography than normal males (Kant & Goldstein, 1970).

What these misconceptions tend to do is to shift the responsibility from the offender to something outside of him. This is what the offender himself does. He projects the responsibility for his own behavior onto external objects like liquor, drugs, the dress and behavior of his victim, pornography —anywhere but where it really belongs. What he cannot face is that he has serious psychological handicaps that lead him, under certain situations, to rape.

Another common misconception regarding the treatment of rapists is that castration is the solution. Even if castration always rendered the individual sexually impotent, which it does not, it certainly would not solve the underlying conflicts and problems in the individual that prompted the assault. His anger and rage will continue to find behavioral outlets, if not in rape than in other forms of physical violence, such as assault and battery, homicide, and suicide.

Incarceration of the convicted rapist temporarily removes him from the street, but a prison term is not effective in rehabilitating him psychologically. Since prison terms have a maximum limit, and rapists are seldom given a life sentence unless they kill their victim, there will come a time when the offender will be returned to society without any assurance that he no longer constitutes a danger to the community. As a sensible alternative to imprisonment, a number of states[4] have developed a special mental health facility to which a convicted sex offender may be committed indefinitely in lieu of or in addition to a prison sentence. In such programs, any person who is likely to repeat his sexual assaults is quarantined in what must be a humane environment. While hospitalized, the offender can be treated by a range of therapeutic modalities, such as chemotherapy, psychotherapy (individual, group, family, milieu, etc.), behavior modification, and psychoeducational courses (sex education, assertiveness training, etc.), in an effort to bring to bear the mental health professions' knowledge of human behavior on those personality defects that operate in the offender to jeopardize the safety of others. Only in this way can society be protected. The offender should not be released to the community while he continues to be a risk to others. At the same time, once he has been rehabilitated, he may return to society without having to fulfill a specified but meaningless period of institutionalization.

Rape is a serious social problem that has been ignored until recently.

[4]California, Colorado, Florida, Indiana, Maryland, Massachusetts, Minnesota, Missouri, New Jersey, New Mexico, Pennsylvania, Washington, and Wisconsin.

Through the relatively new study of forensic psychology, we are beginning to develop a better understanding of sexual offenders. Perhaps, we have begun to dispel some of the misconceptions about rape. Although these misconceptions are comforting in their simplicity, they lead us to adopt ineffective preventive measures and thus to perpetuate the danger that this form of sexual pathology poses to the community.

Having for so long regarded rape as a symptom of evil to be punished or as an act of sexual brashness to be excused, we have now begun to realize that it is in fact a symptom of psychological dysfunction. Perhaps at long last, the stereotypes of the sexual offender are beginning to give way to the more accurate impression of him as a dangerously troubled man.

Reference

Kant, H. S., & Goldstein, M. J. Pornography. *Psychology Today* (December 1970).

3

Rape Typology and the Coping Behavior of Rape Victims

ANN WOLBERT BURGESS AND
LYNDA LYTLE HOLMSTROM

To understand rape from the victim's point of view, we spent a year talking with all rape victims admitted to the emergency floors of the Boston City Hospital. It became clear in our conversations that rape is an act initiated by the assailant, and that it is not primarily a sexual act but an act of violence. We learned that it was very important to the victims how their assailants gained access to them, that is, the mode of attack. We therefore analyzed all these cases, whether adult, adolescent, or child victims, and we developed a typology of rape based on the assailant's method of attack. The two main styles were (1) the blitz rape and (2) the confidence rape.

Victims of rapists are either singled out for a sudden surprise attack or tricked into trusting the assailant as in any confidence game. In both inci-

ANN WOLBERT BURGESS, R.N., D.N.Sc. ● Director of Nursing Research, School of Nursing, Boston University, Boston, Massachusetts; Chairperson, Rape Prevention and Control Advisory Committee, U.S. Department of Health, Education and Welfare.   LYNDA LYTLE HOLMSTROM, Ph.D. ● Professor and Chairperson, Department of Sociology, Boston College, Boston, Massachusetts.

The section on rape typology is adapted with the permission of the Robert J. Brady Co. from Chapter 1 in *Rape: Victims of Crisis* by Ann W. Burgess and Lynda L. Holmstrom, (Bowie, Md.: Robert J. Brady Co., 1974); pp. 4–11. The section on the coping behavior of the rape victim is reprinted with permission of the *American Journal of Psychiatry* and copyrighted by American Psychiatric Association from "Coping Behavior of the Rape Victim" by Ann W. Burgess and Lynda L. Holmstrom, *American Journal of Psychiatry, 133* (4 April 1976), 413–417.

dences, the sexual act is performed by force or threat of force and without the victim's consent.

The blitz rape occurs suddenly without warning and without prior interaction between assailant and victim. In this sort of rape, the victim is going about her life as usual when suddenly she is seized by the assailant. From her point of view, there is no ready explanation for the man's presence. He suddenly appears, uninvited, and forces himself into the situation. Often, he selects an anonymous victim and tries to remain anonymous himself. He may wear a mask or gloves or cover the victim's face as he attacks.

The typical example of the blitz type of rape occurs when a woman happens to cross the path of the assailant who is looking for someone to capture and attack.

The surprise attack outdoors is classified as a common blitz type of rape. However, it is not unusual for the victim to be attacked while she is asleep in her own bed by an assailant who has gained entry.

> A 62-year-old woman was brought to the hospital at 8:30 A.M. by the police. She had multiple bruises on her face, neck, chest, and back, as well as a two-inch stab wound in her abdomen. Her first words to the counselor were "I thought I was going to be killed. I didn't want to die —I didn't think it was my time, but I remember thinking this is the way I was going to die." The victim said that she had been in her bed sleeping. It was around 3 A.M., and she woke up to feel someone jumping on her. She said, "I started screaming and he put a blanket over my head. I didn't have it off till he left. He said when he started, 'Let's see how you like this.' He started doing such crazy things. He was playing with my breasts and then he made me open my mouth and he put his thing in it. I never did such a thing. He made me keep my hands away from my mouth and he stuck it down so far I thought I would gag. It was just awful. Then he turned me over and tried my back end. He kept turning me this way and that. He raped me the regular way. At least he wasn't violent doing that: thank heaven that wasn't crazy. . . . I remember thinking that I never thought such a thing could happen to me. I thought I would die, and his hand kept clamping my neck tighter and tighter. When he finished raping me, he told me to keep the blanket over my head for 20 minutes and said if I took the blanket off, he would finish me. I didn't hear him leave, but every now and then, I would call out to see if he was still there. I hoped to get a view of him and kept peeking out of the blanket, but I couldn't see anything. Finally, I dared to take the blanket off and I called the police. They came right away and I called my daughter. The officer talked to my daughter and said I was lucky to be alive. I could hardly talk and was having a lot of trouble breathing." The victim was unable to identify an assailant, although she did work with the police in hopes of finding a suspect. She definitely would have pressed charges against the assailant.

The children and adolescents who were victims of the blitz rape were often walking home from school, walking home from a friend's house, or playing with neighborhood friends when the attack occurred. The following report is a case in point:

> A 13-year-old victim stated, "It was 9 P.M. and I left my house to go to the corner store for a cupcake and a Coke. I had my portable radio with me. As I was coming home, a guy grabbed me and dragged me down a hill that is in my own yard. . . . He said a lot of nasty things to me and dirty things like was this the first time I fucked? and did I like it? and then he wanted my name and phone number." The assailant made her take her clothes off and then forced her to lie down on her coat; he put a sleeve across her face so she could not see him. The girl said, "He did it three times and he made me kiss him." The victim was noticeably upset with this part and looked as though she would vomit. She said she had tried to scream and struggle but no one heard her. She thought he was a "crazy man" and that "he will be looking for other girls to rape." The assailant ran off, and the girl ran into her home and told her parents, who immediately called the police. The family worked with the police, but a suspect was never found.

The confidence rape is more subtle than the blitz rape. The confidence rape is an attack in which the assailant gains access to the victim under false pretenses by using deceit, then betrayal, and often violence. Characteristically, in this sort of rape there is prior acquaintance between the victim and the assailant, however brief. The assailant may know the victim from some other time and place and thus already have developed some kind of relationship with her, or he may establish a nonthreatening interaction as a prelude to attack. Establishing this nonthreatening relationship might involve a lot of conversation between the victim and the assailant. Like the confidence man, he encourages her to trust him, and then he betrays this trust.

There are variations of this sexual confidence game. When the assailant is a stranger to the intended victim, he will make an effort to strike up a conversation with the woman and to use verbal means to capture her rather than physical force. The assailant establishes a kind of relationship with the victim, ostensibly for a reason acceptable to the victim. For example, the assailant may present himself to his victim as the person who could rescue her from danger:

> A 21-year-old woman was walking home from work. She saw two men behind her, one on foot and one on a motorbike. The man on the motorbike approached her and convinced her that the man on foot was following her and might try to attack her. She was persuaded to accept a ride from him to the square, where she could get a cab. Instead of going to the square, he made several turns on side streets and took her behind a restaurant, where he pushed her down to the ground and took

her clothes off. The woman said, "I cried all through it until he told me I had to stop or he'd hurt me." The police arrived on the scene as the man was trying to escape, having received a call from someone who heard the screams.

A number of people may be involved in the confidence style of attack, either as assailants or as accomplices in the crime. Often another woman serves as a decoy who deceives and entraps the victim. In cases involving hitchhiking victims, there may be a woman sitting in the car alone; the victim-to-be sees that she will get in next to a woman and thinks it will be a safe ride. Women have also deceived the victim in cases of gang rape by making the victim think she was going to a party. Once at the "party," the decoy woman disappears, and the victim very quickly realizes that she is the mark for sexual assault:

> A 29-year-old divorced woman was at a club where people were talking and mingling. The woman was with a group of several men and another woman when the talk focused on a party that was being held that evening. One man suggested they all go to the party. The two men and two women went in one car. They arrived at the apartment, and the victim-to-be went in first, followed by one of the men. The minute she stepped into the apartment, she realized something was wrong when she saw many men standing around with motorcycle jackets on and drinking beer. There were no other women there, and she suddenly realized that the other woman had disappeared. She panicked and said, "This isn't what I expected. I do not wish to stay. Please let me out."
>
> The men did not listen to her. She was pushed into a bathroom, where a man was urinating. When he finished, he forced her to have oral sex, and then she was pushed back out into the room with the other men. Over a two-day period, she was held captive and forced to comply with the sexual demands of eight men and was assaulted if she refused. The sexual demands were for oral sex, during which time the men ejaculated in her mouth, and anal and vaginal sex, with several men demanding sexual acts simultaneously.
>
> The victim feared that she might be murdered. She was taken by car to a second apartment in another town during part of the orgy. She was released when her purse was examined and it was learned that she worked for a local personality.

There are many attacks where the assailant is known to the victim. The assailant is a neighbor, an acquaintance, a date, a friend, or a relative. The assailant uses his relationship with the victim to trick her into allowing him an opportunity to attack her:

> A 19-year-old woman was brought to the emergency ward by the police one evening at 1:30 A.M. She was tearful and said, "I am shocked that this happened. I cannot understand it; he has a girlfriend; how

could he do such a thing?" The young woman went on to say that this had been her wedding day and that she and her husband were at their wedding reception. Her husband had become angry at one of the guests who he felt was paying too much attention to her, and that prompted him to leave her. The bride then went looking for her husband. An invited guest, a friend of the groom, said that he would help find the groom, saying that he knew where he was. The bride left with the friend, who said that the groom was across the street, and as they headed toward the place, the friend forced the woman against the wall and held something to her throat that felt like a knife. The man said, "I want you and I am going to have you." The victim said, "He tried to do it standing up but couldn't. He then forced me to lie down on the ground, and he took off my pants and raped me lying down." When the man finished, he took off down the street. The victim said that she became hysterical and ran into a stranger who asked what happened. He listened and then they went to a nearby restaurant and called the police.

A large number of assailants of adolescents and children know their victim prior to the attack. The assailant could be a school peer, known casually to the girl, who suddenly attacks her on the way home from school. Often this is a gang rape involving several youths and one girl:

A 13-year-old girl reported, "We were at the sub shop. There were four of us—my girl friend and two boys we knew from school. The boys suggested going to this building to play games. I said yes; I thought it would be fun. I thought we would play pool. We went there, went up in the elevator and into the room through a sliding window. I thought it was a settlement house where all the kids go. . . . In the room, he kissed me. I told him to stop, that I wasn't that kind of girl. He used one hand to hold my arms together. . . . He was undressing me with his other hand. We fought. He punched me. I punched him back in the mouth. I got a bruised finger because of it. He said to let him do it or he'd stick it in hard. He said he wouldn't let me go till he checked to see if I was a virgin. . . . Then he got on top of me. He attacked me."

There are situations where the primary motive of rape is to control the woman over a long period of time. The woman is frequently an ex-girlfriend of the assailant, who assumes that he still has full sexual privileges with her. The victim is beaten as well as sexually assaulted. A 45-year-old woman was the victim in this situation:

The woman arrived at the emergency ward at 3:30 A.M. accompanied by her boyfriend. She said the man who assaulted her had been a previous boyfriend of hers for a one-and-a-half-year period and that he had come to her apartment uninvited that evening. She said, "Men should not be allowed to get away with this kind of thing. Most women do not press charges. They are so frightened they will be killed if they do tell. And many women end up dead in an apartment from such a thing and no one knows what has happened to them. Well, I am going to tell on this guy. He gave me a shakedown. He knew where to hit me and how to get me scared so I would do what he told me, and I did. . . . He said he'd beat me if I tell. And he gave me a sample tonight to show me. You know, they work you over—to control you—so they can have you sexually any time they want."

The woman went to the police station the next day to report the assault. She identified the man. The police never arrested the man but suggested that she file the complaint as a civil complaint. When she was asked how she felt about her experience with the legal process, the woman said, "I decided to relax on it. He said he would deny it and say he didn't do it. He said I'd be ashamed to bring such a thing out in the open—said what would my family and friends think. He just would deny the whole thing. But I have something on him and he will get what he deserves. . . . I am just one more poor little victim who is helpless, and he is an untouchable because of who he is and who he works for. It is not so much outsmarting these men but being lucky enough to survive. As long as I know he is not bothering me, I feel okay. I have pointed him out to my friends so that they know him, and I am covered for future experiences."

There are adolescents and children who are controlled in this way, too. The victim feels unable to tell family or anyone else about the assaults. The assailant trades on this fear and continues to molest or assault the child. In such situations, the child or adolescent is manipulated by the assailant over time:

A 17-year-old male babysitter terrorized six children in a family, both boys and girls, over a one-year period. The assailant would select one of the oldest children to molest sexually until the victim was able to resist him physically. He would then select the next oldest child. The oldest girl, age 9, was able to verbally fight off the assailant, who said that he "didn't like girls." The assailant threatened physical harm to the children if they told anyone what he was doing.

The experience of rape varies with the modus operandi of the rapist and the reactions of the victim. In the preceding section of this chapter, we formulated a behavioral typology of rape from the victim's viewpoint, based on how the assailant gains access to the victim. The mode of attack has important implications for how the victims cope in the attack situation.

There have been several recent studies of victim crisis situations involving major crimes, including forcible rape and situations in which victims have successfully interrupted or prevented attack (Burgess & Holmstrom, 1974; Schultz, 1975; Queens Bench Foundation, 1975). Giacenti and Tjaden (1973) reported that out of 915 cases in the Denver area, 319 victims were able to interrupt the rape by active resistance, fleeing, physically fighting, crying aloud, verbal refusals, and outside intervention.

We found it useful to study the victim's coping behavior at three points relative to the attack: during the early awareness of danger, during the attack itself, and after the attack. Most of the victims we interviewed perceived the rape, whether blitz or confidence rape, as a life-threatening experience. The minority who did not fear for their lives still saw the rape as an acutely stressful, frightening, and degrading experience. For almost all victims, this attack was something far out of the ordinary that seriously taxed their adaptive resources.

Appraisal of the degree of danger, threat, or harm is a psychological process that intervenes between a stressful event and coping behavior. This early awareness may be cognitive, perceptual, or affective—often, the victim describes it as a "sixth sense" or a feeling of impending danger. The coping task during this phase is to react quickly to this warning.

Only 15 of the 92 women we interviewed spontaneously reported some cognitive or perceptual awareness of the potential danger they faced, and they were not totally clear about the nature of the danger; they just knew that something was wrong. Reports of this vague, obscurely formulated consciousness of danger varied. Victims said that they saw a strange man and either thought he might do harm, wondered why he had been hanging around all evening, remembered seeing him before, looked at the car that pulled up, thought it strange that the apartment light did not go on, or heard a noise in the kitchen and went to investigate.

The threat of attack is the point when the person realizes that there is definite danger to his or her life. The coping task at this stage is to attempt to avoid or escape the danger. The person is aware that something critical is going to happen but may not realize that rape is the imminent danger; for example, the person may instead fear robbery or aggravated assault.

Coping behavior was analyzed in terms of whether or not victims were able to react to the confrontation with danger. This ability to react often depended on the amount of time between the threat of attack and the attack, on the type of attack, and on the type of force or violence used.

A majority of the victims used one or more strategies, and a minority of the victims were unable to use any strategies (see Table 1). We have divided the basic strategies into three categories: cognitive assessment, verbal tactics, and physical action. Victims may cope by cognitively assessing the situation to determine possible alternatives; for example, they may think about how they can get away from the assailant's grasp or escape from a car or room safely, or they may worry that the man will panic and hurt them and plan how to keep calm. Their assessment may lead to a verbal or physical strategy of action or result in no action at all.

Victims may cope verbally, as the majority of our sample did, by trying to *talk their way out of the situation* ("I tried to engage them in conversation, such as asking where they went to school and why they were doing this"); *stall for time* ("I tried to talk to him; tried to get him to come for coffee at a restaurant down the street"); _reason with the assailant by trying to change his mind_ ("I'm a married woman"; "I'm a virgin"); _gain sympathy from the assailant_ ("Look at the trouble you're causing me"; "What will I do?"); _use flattery_ ("You're an attractive man; surely you don't have to do this for sex"); _bargain with the assailant_ ("There's my TV; take it and go"); _feign illness_ ("I'm sick"); _threaten the assailant_ ("My husband is due home"; "My kids are in the next room"; "A policeman lives in this building"); _retaliate verbally_ ("Get your hands off me"; "Don't touch me"; "What are you doing?"); _change the assailant's perception of the victim_ ("I talked to him like a mother"); _joke or trick him into leaving_ (a woman awakes to see a man coming into her room saying, "I'm escaping from the police"; she says, "Okay—I'll let you out the back door").

One-third of the victims were unable to use any strategy to avoid the attack. The victim might be physically paralyzed and totally overpowered by the assailant. For example, several victims were in their beds sleeping when the assailant gained access to their apartments and attacked them ("It was around 3 A.M. . . . I woke to feel someone jumping on me"). The victim might be walking down the street and suddenly grabbed by one or two assailants. The use of a weapon often paralyzed a person. The following example from a referral case illustrates early awareness of danger followed by physical paralysis: "The door buzzer rang. I was expecting friends and opened my door . . . saw three men with a paper in one's hand. . . . I froze . . . paralyzed for a moment . . . something went through my head . . . shut the door but they pushed it back open . . . with the gun. . . ." In some cases, the victim was totally stunned or surprised by the change in behavior of a man whom she knew as a friend, a neighbor, or an acquaintance and said "He just grabbed me before I knew it."

Victims may be psychologically paralyzed either through their defensive structure ("When I realized what he was going to do, I blanked out . . . tried not to be aware of what was going on") or because of their use of

Table 1. Coping Behavior of 92 Rape Victims in Response to Threat of Attack

Description of behavior	Number of victims
Victims with strategies ($N = 58$)[a]	
Cognitive assessment	18
Verbal tactics	57
Physical action	21
Victims without strategies ($N = 34$)	
Physically paralyzed	22
Psychologically paralyzed	12

[a]Many victims had more than one strategy; therefore, the total numbers exceed 58.

alcohol or drugs prior to the attack. Thoughts of death may paralyze a victim ("I thought he'd be the last person I'd see alive").

Physical action aimed at preventing the assault by fleeing from the situation or fighting the assailant was a strategy used by 21 women in our sample. Most often physical action was used in combination with verbal resistance, but in some cases, it was the primary strategy ("I tried to stab him with the broken glass"; "I tried to push him back out of the apartment").

Of our sample, 31 women used multiple strategies to avoid the rape; 27 used one; and 34 used none. One woman who was successful in avoiding attack said, "First I tried to calm him down; tried to talk softly to him and said, 'Okay, we'll be friends.' Then I said my brother was due home any time. . . . I tried all I knew, verbal and physical. . . . I screamed and fought. . . ." The brother did come home, and the assailant left without completing the rape.

Another victim who tried several strategies was not successful. Three men forced her into a car as she waited for a bus after her evening classes at a local university. She tried verbal tactics ("My husband will be worried and probably call the police if I am not home"), but the assailants told her that such remarks would "get me dead." The victim then became silent. She later tried bargaining ("I offered them my money to let me go") and finally decided to comply ("I decided the only way was to play it their way").

In another case, one can see the coping behaviors of early awareness, an affective reaction of fear, cognitive assessment, and verbal tactics of joking: "I got a warning . . . saw two men at the end of my hall . . . got frightened . . . didn't know how they got there. They said they needed to

Table 2. Coping Behavior of 90 Women during Rape

Description of behavior	Number of victims
Cognitive strategies	28
Affective response ($N = 25$)	
Crying	17
Anger	8
Verbal Strategies ($N = 23$)	
Screaming	14
Talking	9
Physical action	23
Psychological defense	17
Physiological reaction	10
No strategy	1
No data	8

use my phone. I tried to joke and said, 'Who you trying to call, Red China?''

If initial strategies to escape fail, there is a point in the attack situation when it becomes clear to the victim that forced sexual assault is unavoidable. The coping task during this phase is to survive the rape despite the many demands forced upon the victim, such as oral, vaginal, and anal penetration. She may also be forced to have conversation with the assailant. Victims coped with the actual rape in a variety of ways, as Table 2 indicates.

Victims often cope during the rape itself by mentally focusing and directing their attention to some specific thought to distance themselves from the reality of the event. Remaining calm may be used as a strategy of survival during which the woman focuses on controlling her reactions so as not to provoke additional violence. The victim might talk to herself, as in the following case:

> I kept thinking keep cool. He said he'd kill me. He hit me, he choked me, he could kill me. I said to myself, "You can handle anything; come on, you can do it." I decided not to fight him . . . he was holding my neck so tight. . . . I responded a little to him . . . that blew his mind that I acted as I did. It was very quick, thank God.

Memorizing details was a strategy that paid off later in some cases. One victim said, "I focused on their faces and thought to myself, 'I'll see you guys in court if I get out of this alive.' " She did. Another victim said, "I played detective . . . tried to observe everything, like the tattoo on his arm, remarks he made, route of travel of the car, license of the car."

Recalling advice people have given on the subject of rape is another coping mechanism victims report: "I remember a conversation I had with my husband. He said if I was attacked not to resist if he wants sex. My husband said the guy could kill me or the children . . . but sex wouldn't kill me." Another victim said, "I remember talking with people about rape, and they always said not to resist . . . that a female could be killed, beaten, or mutilated. I didn't want that to happen."

Memories of previous violent situations determined the behavior of some victims ("I struggled a little . . . then remembered when I was 12 I fought a neighbor boy and got my nose broken"). Praying for help was used as a tactic to decrease stress and tension ("I wasn't listening to them but concentrating on praying that my friends who had keys to my apartment would come"). Concentrating on the assailant in terms of who he was and what had led to this attack was also a strategy ("I remember thinking that this person must have a home—must live somewhere . . . why would he do this on Mother's Day? . . . I thought of the irony of it."). Compliance was a strategy used to "speed it up . . . get it over with." To many victims, the attack seemed interminable.

Victims combined verbal and affective responses by screaming and yelling. This tactic served both to relieve tension and to deter the assailant from his full intent. Screams brought police to the scene in several cases, which sometimes resulted in the assailant's being apprehended during the attack.

Several victims believed that talking with the assailant during the rape helped them avoid additional violence. The assailant may demand to know how the victim is "enjoying" the rape. One victim handled the situation as follows: "He kept wanting to know if it felt good and I had to say yes to keep him happy. . . . He said, 'I'm on drugs lady and I need money . . . fuck me good or I'll kill you.' He needed to be reassured."

If the attack continues over a period of time, the victim may try verbal tactics to calm the assailant and thus avoid further demands ("I talked to calm him down. . . . I asked questions and he kept talking"). Sarcasm may be used as a coping strategy, especially if that is the victim's usual verbal style.

> As he was molesting me, he asked if I enjoyed it and I said, 'Oh sure, it is great." I decided to go along with him. He seemed to need reassurance . . . I wasn't scared then. First thought he'd get his kicks and then it'd be all over—I'd be dead. I got faith that he wasn't going to harm me.

Some victims tried to gain control of the situation by scaring the assailant(s) ("You'll be in real trouble if you kill me"; "You'll be sorry. . . . I'll get someone to kill you"). This strategy was partially successful in some cases.

Some victims reported physically resisting penetration ("I struggled and tightened my muscles"). Sometimes the victim struggled to a certain point and then stopped ("I fought and struggled until I realized he was going to rape me. He wanted to rape me more than I could manage to resist"). Some victims quickly discovered that struggling and fighting were just what the assailant wanted ("The more I screamed and fought, the more excited he would get").

In addition to behavioral reactions, internal defense mechanisms are used to cope psychologically with the fear produced during the attack. Some women denied the experience ("I never thought it could happen"); others experienced dissociative feelings ("I pinched myself to see if I was real"); others suppressed the rape ("I am missing 10 minutes of my life"); while others rationalized the situation ("I felt sorry for him if this was the only way he knew how to get sex"). One victim described her reaction as follows: "I did not struggle because of the knife. All those things you read about or plan to do don't help. . . . I felt I was not going to get out alive. . . . I was resigned; I felt nothing, empty; felt this can't happen to me."

Not all coping behavior is voluntary and conscious. Certainly, some screaming and yelling is involuntary, and victims also reported physiological responses of choking, gagging, nausea, vomiting, pain, urinating, hyperventilating, and losing consciousness. One victim described an epileptic seizure:

> Only thing I remember is getting the key into the lock to get into the building. Then I got warning signs to my seizure attacks . . . getting overheated and the ringing in my ears and that's all. When I regained consciousness, I was in the hall by the door to the basement. I dragged myself out as I heard someone saying, "Who left their keys in the door?"

Another victim described how her involuntary reaction scared the assailant away after he raped her: "I felt faint, trembling and cold. . . . I went limp. I think he got scared and thought I was out."

The stressful situation is not over for the victim when the actual rape ends. She must alert others to her distress, escape from the assailant, or free herself from where she has been left. Victims are always hopeful that someone will come to their aid, and they may spend time concentrating on how to obtain help. In one case, the victim's coping behavior after the attack was complicated by the response of the police.

> After he left, I felt stunned and immobilized lying there on the sidewalk. . . . My mind was racing and I tried to decide what to do. I got up because I thought he might try to come back . . . told the officers and they said, "Another rape? Sorry lady, we're busy" and drove off. . . . I was enraged and started crying . . . ran home and pulled the telephone plug from the wall . . . felt I couldn't talk with anyone . . . then took a bath and sat there till the water was freezing.

In this case, the victim's initial reaction was physical immobilization, yet her mind was very active. Her crisis request for police intervention was ignored, and this rejection depleted her coping strength, allowing her only an affective response of anger and tears. Fleeing to the safety of her apartment, she immediately isolated herself from all outside contact and sought the comfort of a bath.

Often the victim must negotiate with the assailant for her release. The assailant sometimes apologizes and tries to gain sympathy and thus get the victim to promise not to tell, or he may give the victim orders or instructions ("I'll kill you if you tell or go to the police"; "Don't move from that position for 30 minutes"). During this bargaining process the victim may cope by remaining silent or agreeing to instructions. Some victims promised not to tell anyone or invented stories to preserve their lives: "I told him my girlfriend had this happen, and when she went to the police, they didn't believe her. I told him I'd never go to the police."

If the victim has been tied and gagged, she has to cope with physically freeing herself ("I lay still for a moment . . . then realized that the faster I got myself untied, the faster I could get to the police and my friends . . . ankle ties . . . getting cramps in my legs . . . so I had to tell myself not to panic and I worked the wrist ties and ankle ties next").

The stress period of actual danger ends when the victim is free from her assailant and is returned to a safe place. Mastery, in terms of survival, may be verbalized by the victim as well as by her family and friends: "The worst is over. . . I got through it. . . . I am grateful to survive." Appreciation of the fact that the victim has successfully managed to survive a life-threatening assault is a positive beginning to the long-term process of coping with the aftermath of the rape.

Crisis intervention aimed at assisting women with the stress following a rape must be based on awareness of the coping strategies employed during the rape.

Rapoport (1962) noted that patterns of coping in crisis situations may be adaptive or maladaptive. Parad and Resnik (1975) stated that the purpose of actively focused crisis intervention is to steer the person toward adaptive coping and away from maladaptive behavior. Adams and Lindemann (1974) formulated coping principles drawn from a study of catastrophic disabling injuries; they emphasized identifying the acute crisis and the psychological means by which the crisis is to be managed, if not mastered.

Assessment of the victim's coping behavior provides the counselor with two therapeutic measures. First, during the onset and duration of the assault, acknowledgment of the woman's coping strategies can be used as a supportive measure. By listening to the victim recount the rape, clinicians can identify specific coping behavior and label it as such for the victim. This approach tells victims that their behavior functioned as a positive adaptive mechanism to allow them to survive a life-threatening situation. By conveying this information, the counselor attempts to alleviate some of the guilt suffered by a victim, who may think, "I did not do enough—I could have done more." This approach reinforces a positive sense of self-esteem and worth. As was noted by one victim, who was raped by two assailants at knife point, "At least I wasn't so whacked out that I couldn't get a description and license of the car." Reaffirming the strategic use of her cognitive abilities helped this victim to see herself as a person who was able to do something in a highly stressful situation, even though she was physically immobilized. Identifying coping strategies strengthens the therapeutic alliance in terms of providing positive expectations regarding the victim's capacity to restore herself to her precrisis level of functioning. Murphy's model of resilience (1974), wherein a person sees herself as someone who is resilient and expects to recover from the trauma, has significance in counseling rape victims and fostering active mastery of stress.

The second use of the assessment of coping behavior during the assault is to give the counselor a reference point from which to begin the clinical negotiation for crisis service (Burgess & Lazare, 1976). For example, one request may be related to primary prevention in terms of what other strategies might be used in such situations. The clinician can explore with the victim the crisis behaviors she used and analyze their effectiveness. New strategies might be suggested as possibilities in future stressful situations. It is important to help expand the person's problem-solving capabilities (Hamburg & Adams, 1967).

We believe that our analysis of the coping behavior of rape victims opens up many other research areas. Perhaps the most important question is: Can specific victim coping behaviors be matched with specific assailant modes of attack to identify and/or maximize those tactics that result in the least amount of victim trauma, both during and after the encounter?

References

Adams, J. E., & Lindemann, E. Coping with long-term disability. In G., Coelho, D. Hamburg, & J. Adams, (Eds.), *Coping and adaptation*. New York: Basic Books, 1974, pp. 127–138.

Burgess, A. W., & Holmstrom, L. L. *Rape: Victims of crisis*. Bowie, Md.: Robert J. Brady Company, 1974.

Burgess, A. W., & Lazare, A. *Community mental health: Target populations*. Englewood Cliffs, N.J.: Prentice-Hall, 1976.

Giacenti, T. A., & Tjaden, C. The crime of rape in Denver. Denver, Colo.: Denver High Impact Anticrime Council (unpublished report), 1973.

Hamburg, D. A., & Adams, J. E. A perspective on coping behavior. *Archives of General Psychiatry*, 1967, *17*, 277–284.

Murphy, L. B. Coping, vulnerability and resilience in childhood. In G. Coelho, D. Hamburg, & J. Adams (Eds.), *Coping and adaptation*. New York: Basic Books, 1974, pp. 69–100.

Parad, H. J., & Resnik, H. L. P. The practice of crisis intervention in emergency care. In H. L. P. Resnik, & H. L. Ruben, (Eds.), *Emergency psychiatric care*. Bowie, Md.: Charles Press, 1975, pp. 23–34.

Queens Bench Foundation. Rape victimization study. San Francisco, Calif.: Queens Bench Foundation, 1975.

Rapoport, L. The state of crisis: Some theoretical considerations. *Social Services Review*, 1962, *36*, 211–217.

Schultz, L. G. (Ed.). *Rape victimology*. Springfield, Ill.: Charles C Thomas, 1975.

II

The Hospital Emergency Room

Many victims come to a hospital emergency room following a rape. Because of injury and the risk of venereal disease and pregnancy, women who may not report the rape to the police or confide in friends and family do turn to the hospital for assistance. The victim's experience in the emergency room can influence her subsequent decisions about reporting the crime and seeking further help. Since hospital personnel are commonly the first community members to come in contact with a woman after a rape, their behavior and attitudes are frequently taken by the victim as indicators of the kind of reception she can expect from others. If she is treated with respect and concern, she is more likely to be accessible to further assistance, be it from police, friends, or professionals.

We firmly believe that every hospital has the ethical responsibility to develop a plan for the treatment of rape victims commensurate with their resources and their community needs. Each hospital has different capabilities and serves different kinds of communities. Smaller suburban or rural hospitals may need to devise a plan for triage and transportation to one facility designated to offer a full rape treatment program. Regional medical care planning is called for to avoid unnecessary duplication of services and at the same time to ensure that adequate treatment is readily accessible. The cooperation of other community agencies, such as social service or mental health facilities and volunteer women's crisis groups, must be elicited by the hospital to ensure referral resources for services they cannot provide. Liaison with local police, state crime laboratories, and district attorney's offices is crucial in securing their input for protocols to adequately cover evidence collection and medical–legal procedures. Once a protocol for rape treatment is established, it is equally important for the hospital to inform the community of the availability of service, since too many victims are deprived of medical care because of ignorance of existing resources.

This section covers the emergency room treatment of the rape victim. It is intended to be a guide for nurses and emergency room physicians in particular and to familiarize counselors, police, and lawyers with the medical procedures in rape cases.

The chapter by Barbara Schuler Gilmore and Janet Weeks Evans details the pivotal role of the nurse both as a clinician and as the coordinator of staff teaming in the emergency room. They recommend a primary nursing model. Their discussion includes a review of the emotional responses of the nurse to this particular patient population and the ways in which certain behaviors can either increase or reduce their effectiveness with the victim. Integration of medical, legal, social, and psychological concerns is emphasized in their holistic approach to the victim. In addition to clinical guidelines, Gilmore and Evans point out the necessity for intra-hospital liaison among various departments and disciplines (such as pathology and gynecology) and liaison with community resources (such as the police, mental health agencies, and volunteer groups). The nurse may be the best and, in some hospitals, the only person able to coordinate the interdisciplinary cooperation needed to provide comprehensive treatment.

Henry Klapholz's chapter concentrates on the physician's role and the medical treatment of the victim. He explains the proper history, examination, and treatment for rape victims and underscores the importance of the physician's sensitivity to the psychic trauma of his patient. He refers to the need for careful, detailed, and *legible* documentation of history, observations, and findings in the patient's medical record for possible future use in court. Additional description of evidence collection in the emergency room is presented in Chapter 6, "The Police Investigation," and in the nursing and medical guidelines included in the appendix.

4

The Nursing Care of Rape Victims

Barbara Schuler Gilmore and Janet Weeks Evans

Every case of rape is unique. For this reason, emergency unit (EU) nursing services, along with other health care and legal systems, have begun to develop guidelines to provide appropriate individualized care for victims. With new appreciation of the effects of this violent crime, it is evident that the emergency care following a rape has tremendous impact on the victim. Sensitive, thorough, and informed nursing contributes in a major way to assuring that this impact is in support of the victim's ability to cope (Appell, Baskin, & Smith, 1976; Klingbeil, Anderson, & Vontver, 1976).

EU nursing care is determined by a holistic perspective of the victim. This view includes attention to immediate emotional and physical needs, to the social aspects of the victim's plight, to immediate and long-range legal concerns, and to possible referral of the victim to resource persons with expertise in these areas and in the prevention of long-term physical and psychological problems. All of these factors contribute to the long-term goal of the victim's return to a state of health and well-being.

Achieving these goals and providing optimal care for the victim is a challenge because of the nature of the assault and the emotions it evokes. It requires that the nurse who deals primarily with physical illness and injury be able to call on her equally important but less visible skill of responding to the person suffering intense emotional trauma. The ability to be supportive and reassuring despite one's own strong emotions evoked by the victim's situation comes with self-knowledge, experience, maturity, and an acquired sensitivity to the unique trauma that is rape.

Another difficulty is the locale in which the care is provided. Most EUs

Barbara Schuler Gilmore, R.N., M.S.N. ● Coordinator, Rape Service, Newton-Wellesley Hospital, Newton Lower Falls, Massachusetts.   Janet Weeks Evans, R.N. ● Nursing Coordinator, Rape Crisis Intervention Program, Beth Israel Hospital, Boston, Massachusetts.

are busy and unpredictable. They are staffed by many disciplines with different specific functions; the nursing staff is augmented by a variety of on-call physicians and perhaps technicians, students, clerks, housekeepers, and security staff. Add to this a collection of other patients and concerned relatives, and it is apparent that the EU is a very difficult setting in which to provide and coordinate a sensitive care plan for the victim.

In spite of these difficulties, emergency care of victims can be effective. It is the aim of this chapter to review several important considerations that impinge on the nursing aspects of that care. Primary nursing, as opposed to functional nursing, has many advantages as a model of delivering good care to rape victims in an EU. Emotions evoked in the nurse by the experience of dealing with a rape victim are explored because of the part they play in the nurse's response to the victim. The last section deals with in-house and community issues to be considered when evolving an approach to caring for rape victims. An example of an operational nursing protocol is provided in Appendix 1, "Guidelines for the Nursing Care of Rape Victims in the Emergency Unit."

For the sake of expediency, the authors have decided that both nurse and victim will be referred to in the female gender. This is not to imply that all victims or all nurses are female; obviously, they are not. In the same vein, not all rapes are heterosexual; there are also homosexual male rapes and Lesbian rapes. Because of space and time constraints, these will not be addressed specifically. Rather, we have chosen to address what is by far the most common rape situation: a female victim, raped by a man, and cared for by a female nurse. Male nurses will find that Chapter 14 elucidates some of the emotions men experience when dealing with rape victims.

Application of the Primary Nursing Model

In the analysis of the rape victim's needs, the challenge to nursing becomes evident. The complexities of the situation, the variables of victim's age, personality, life experience, and coping ability, plus the specifics of the assault combine to produce a very demanding nursing care problem. Each victim is an individual, and therefore, each responds differently. Because of these factors, primary nursing is the model best suited to the care of the victims.

Primary nursing allows for individualized care planning. The plan is devised by the nurse and the victim in response to the nurse's assessment of the victim's needs. The nurse is responsible not only for assessment and planning but also for implementation through collaboration with members of other disciplines. In the rape victim's case, these are the counselor who will do the crisis intervention with the victim and the gynecologist who will do the physical exam. The primary nurse will also provide the direct nursing care to the victim as indicated. Evaluation of the care and the provision of follow-up planning are also the primary nurse's responsibility. The primary nurse is accountable to the victim for the care provided (Logsdon, 1973).

The essence of primary nursing is in the relationship between nurse and victim. The relationship provides the victim with a consistent, predictable, and trustworthy person (the nurse) who imparts acceptance, understanding, and respect. This is the first effort at repairing and restoring the victim's integrity so recently invaded and undermined.

Via this relationship, the primary nurse and the victim together identify the desired goals. Clearly, the rape has produced terrifying results, *outcomes* in nursing-care-plan parlance. Generally, rape victims experience intense anxiety, fear, loss of control, and varying degrees of physical damage and risk (pregnancy and venereal disease). Modification of these outcomes then becomes the goal of both victim and nurse (Little & Carnevali, 1976).

Expected outcomes and observed responses vary from victim to victim. Reduction of anxiety and fear will be demonstrated by a decrease in the victim's behavioral demonstrations of anxiety and fear—for example, shaking, trembling, crying, and handwringing—as well as by being able to talk about the decreased feelings. Loss of control is an issue for anyone needing emergency care. There is the obvious risk that the feelings of helplessness sustained by the victim during the assault could be compounded during the emergency visit. Restoring control to the victim begins by honoring her crisis request. The mechanism of "informed consent" reinforces that control, and the expected outcome will be her ability to discuss her options and decide what she wants.

Keeping the expected outcomes in mind will influence the primary nurse as she works with the victim. For the rape victim, having one individual to whom to relate will go far to decrease the confusion inherent in the emergency medical situation, in which every new face may be perceived as a potential rapist. The calm, nonjudgmental caring demonstrated by the primary nurse will help to diminish the intense anxiety the victim experiences. Then, the victim's ability to understand the treatment and the reasons for it will be considerably increased. Her understanding will produce a sound basis for the informed consent necessary for treatment and for effective follow-up planning (Hilberman, 1976).

The primary nurse, remaining with the victim during the EU visit, will become sensitive to the victim's individualized response to the trauma and her style of communicating, verbal and nonverbal. "Tuning in," the nurse will learn the particular social, psychological, or physical concerns of the victim (Burgess & Holmstrom, 1973; Manthey, Ciske, Robertson, & Harris, 1970). In addition to the beneficial effects of ventilation for the victim, the nurse can use the information she collects from the victim to facilitate the victim's interaction with other members of the EU team, such as the counselor and the gynecologist. The counselor will be working with the victim around social and psychological issues. The gynecologist will do the physical exam and discuss physical concerns with her. Educating the victim about her legal, medical, and follow-up options will relieve and reassure the victim. Damaging effects of the rape will begin to be undone by placing the control with the victim.

Primary nursing, thorough care planning, and effective communication with team members facilitate the treatment process and ensure the victim of sensitive, comprehensive care.

The Rape Victim in the EU

Sensitive attention to practical details is important in addressing the rape victim. Upon arrival at the EU, the victim should be immediately ushered to a quiet and private room by whichever staff person she first encounters. If any advance notice has been provided, the ideal person to greet her will be the assigned primary nurse. Where advance notice is not available, this assignment must be made quickly, as it has been recommended that the EU give first priority to rape victims just after life-threatening attacks (Brodyaga, Gates, Singer, Tucker, & White, 1975; Hilberman, 1976).

Once assigned, the primary nurse should immediately introduce herself with the brief explanation that she will be with the victim for the entire time that she is in the EU and will explain procedures and answer questions. Her warmth and concern can be actively demonstrated. Offering a cup of coffee may alleviate some of the victim's apprehension and create a feeling of safety.[1] The nurse's verbal reassurances will aid the victim to feel that she is regaining the control so recently lost over her life and body. If the victim has been accompanied to the hospital by friends or family, they should be permitted to remain with the victim if she wants them to do so. As she does the above, the nurse has begun a preliminary assessment of the degree of emotional stress and the physical injuries. The nurse should then ask the woman for a brief description of what happened during the assault, explaining that a more thorough report will be required and recorded when the gynecologist arrives. At this time, the information is needed to effectively treat the most serious problem first.

Initial assessment should be documented on the nursing assessment sheet. Findings and observations should be recorded promptly. Frequently,

[1]Nothing by mouth should be offered if the rapist has ejaculated in the victim's mouth. Sperm or semen if present in the mouth could be used as evidence; also, throat cultures for venereal disease need to be taken if oral penetration has occurred.

an injury such as rope burns around the neck, hands, or feet or strangulation marks caused by the rapist's hands may be very apparent at the onset of the interview but may fade or disappear by the time the patient is given her thorough medical exam.

The mechanics of EU registration should be effected by the primary nurse at some appropriate time. The nurse does this because questions of home address, next of kin, and insurance coverage often stir up fears about confidentiality of treatment. Other concerns are that the rapist may get the victim's home address or that the hospital may automatically notify next of kin. The nurse can deal directly with these legitimate concerns and reassure the victim accordingly. Confidentiality of hospital records can be explained as well as the fact that only at her request or with her consent would anyone be notified of her presence. When this question comes up, it is time for the nurse to discuss with the victim who among family and friends she may want to ask to come and be with her in the EU.

It may fall to the primary nurse to notify these individuals. Before doing so, she should discuss with the victim what others are to be told and then abide by those wishes. The victim is to be supported as she tells significant others. Therefore, the nurse must be available when the family or friends arrive. The calm, accepting, and protective presence of the nurse can provide a model of behavior for the visitor as well as giving the victim encouragement.

At some point during the EU visit, the victim will need to be asked about financial arrangements for billing purposes. This topic should be covered by the primary nurse, who can answer questions and facilitate the procedure in such a way as to decrease the victim's anxiety about arrangements.

The issue of insurance coverage for the EU visit may be complicated. The young woman covered by her parents' family plan may not want her parents to know of the assault. This decision should be respected, and alternative methods of payment should be offered by the hospital. The woman who has her own insurance but who lives at home may prefer that bills be sent to an alternative address. For those women who have no insurance and no money, or a limited income, "free care" or a sliding fee must be considered (Brodyaga et al., 1975).

The primary nurse coordinates interviewing by the police if the victim has chosen to have them involved. During her EU stay, the victim will have increased coping ability if she is not flooded with multiple demands simultaneously. She and the nurse can decide together the most advantageous time to talk with police. Occasionally, law enforcement officials, in their eagerness to pursue the rapist, overwhelm the victim with their need for information. At these times, the primary nurse will have to interrupt the questioning and set limits on the investigators if the victim indicates that she needs a break.

After the preliminary assessment is completed and a care plan has been made with the victim, the primary nurse notifies the team members—that is, the mental health counselor and the gynecologist—in whatever order priorities indicate. Each person should be clearly introduced to the victim so that she has some understanding of who these strangers are and what functions they perform. Whenever possible, the counselor is to be called prior to the gynecological workup, so that the victim has additional support before undergoing what could be construed as a traumatic replay of the rape. Together, the nurse and the counselor should estimate the length of time the victim needs with the counselor before going ahead with the physical exam. Timing is important because the stress of waiting for the exam may cause an increase in anxiety for the victim, making it difficult for her to cooperate.

Physical Examination

When the counselor has finished the interview, the woman should be escorted to the examination room. The nurse explains the physical examination procedures, emphasizing the necessity of a complete examination and full documentation of the assault. Because of the common feelings of helplessness, vulnerability, and fear, it is very important to engage the patient in participating in her care to help restore her sense of control. The patient needs to know what to expect and the reasons for the procedures. Additionally, she needs to know that if at any time the exam is especially difficult for her, she can let the nurse know and they can pause before continuing.

The introduction of the gynecologist should be done prior to positioning for the internal exam. If the size of the hospital physician staff permits, the victim may have the option of a female gynecologist, should she prefer one. However, in most facilities, that option does not exist, and so the presence of the primary nurse is particularly essential as the nurse may be seen as the only reassuring and nonthreatening person in the examining room, the only person capable of empathy at this point.

Discussion with the gynecologist needs to include the findings of the internal exam, an explanation of any damage found, and the recommended treatment. What the woman can expect in terms of pain, tenderness, swelling, bleeding, etc., needs to be addressed. Reassurance on the state of her anatomy is essential. The risk of pregnancy as a result of the rape must be assessed and discussed. The hazards and side effects of medications used for postcoital contraception (pregnancy prevention) must be clearly understood by the victim if she is to be able to give informed consent. She needs to know what options are available should she decide against these drugs and become pregnant. Clear and simple explanations of therapeutic abortion and menstrual extraction, including where they can be obtained, are essential for these women.

✳ The advantages of VD prophylaxis need to be made clear to the victim. Some clinicians feel that the relief the victim experiences at not having to worry about contracting either syphilis or gonorrhea far outweigh the discomfort of the multiple penicillin injections. Victims who opt to "wait and-see" need to understand that an internal exam, on the last day of her next menses, as well as a blood test at that time, will be recommended to diagnose VD. For these reasons it is usually less worrisome for victims to have the prophylactic treatment while in the EU.

For the woman who elects prophylaxis, the primary nurse, being sensitive to the details of the rape, should administer the injections. Requested to turn onto her abdomen, the victim of anal penetration may experience terrifying flashbacks of the rape and may not be able to cooperate with the request. Flexibility as to site of injection and patient positioning is essential. Use of ampicillin capsules could be considered.

When the physical exam has been completed and she is dressed again, having been reassured regarding her internal state, the victim's anxiety level is decreased. She is now more able to understand and discuss treatment and follow-up. This is the time for the nurse to review the treatment and answer questions. The questions may be repeats of those previously answered. When this happens, the victim should not be perceived as stupid or inattentive. Rather, the nurse should remember that high anxiety levels interfere with learning, and thus she should understand the need for repeat explanations.

All explanations need to be made in terms that the patient comprehends. She probably cannot be expected to understand terms like *VD prophylaxis* or *postcoital contraception*. The nurse should anticipate the victim's need for terms that she can understand and substitute accordingly. Veneral disease may have to be discussed in the vernacular, for example, *bad blood,* the *clap.* Postcoital contraception is generally known as the *morning-after pill.*

The high anxiety level is another reason that follow-up counseling is advantageous and should be planned with the victim (Hilberman, 1976). While the victim may feel that everything has been taken care of in the EU, she should be apprised that she may become aware of any number of questions or concerns in the next few days or weeks. It would be comforting for her to know that she has someone with whom she can discuss these things. In hospitals where a counselor is part of the team, the follow-up will probably be offered through the counselor. When a counselor is not part of the medical system, the follow-up, usually telephone counseling, is rightfully part of the primary nurse's responsibility.

Emotional Impact on the Nurse

Much has been written about the emotional responses of victims to rape, but relatively little has been said about the response of the nursing staff who give emergency care to these victims. This area is important because nursing staff must understand how their own emotions may affect their ability to care for the victim.

EU nurses have been raised on the same myths and misconceptions as the general public, and so they respond to rape in many varied emotional ways. This fact indicates the need for continuing education and sensitization programs for EU staff. The object of these programs is to help staff recognize their feelings, understand what they are about, and thus be able to nurse effectively without responding to their own biases or personal reactions (Bellack & Woodard, 1977).

There are several characteristic emotional states that the nurse may experience when caring for victims of sexual assault. The most immediate response the nurse experiences when she hears that a rape victim is coming to the EU is increased *anxiety*. Anxiety prompts people to respond variably, nurses and victims alike. Increased physical activity is one way of dealing with heightened anxiety. The nurse who hurries about assembling equipment, telephoning other members of the team, checking and rechecking the protocol, and running in and out of the victim's room to the degree that she is not available to the victim or her family is responding to her own increased anxiety. The victim could misconstrue the hyperactivity to mean lack of knowledge, inefficiency, or lack of concern. Worse yet, in her shame and mortification, the victim may feel that she is too repulsive for the nurse to stay with. Any of these reactions would be frightening for the victim.

Nurses may respond to increased anxiety by becoming either silent or verbose. The victim may interpret either as disapproval or disinterest and may be prevented from feeling free to vent her feelings or ask questions. The nurse who recognizes her own increased anxiety will be better able to control these behaviors and to respond to the needs of the victim.

Listening to the victim's story, the nurse may also experience increased anxiety if she identifies closely with some portion of the incident. This form of anxiety, dread, is related to a specific danger situation. One EU nurse related the following:

> On a rainy Sunday afternoon last fall, a young woman was brought in by the police. Talking briefly with her, I discovered that she was jumped and raped in a park across from my home. The circumstances were such that whoever had been in that spot at that moment would have been the victim. It could've been me! For the next several days, I was very anxious and nervous when leaving the apartment. I refuse to let my children play in the park.

Nurses may also be reluctant to care for victims because they are concerned (anxious) about talking with them, lest they say the wrong thing and harm the victim further. Genuine statements of concern or reassurance are helpful. Giving information about services and discussing options are also helpful. Being able to listen is very important and one of the most helpful tools available to the nurse. Statements or questions that are not pertinent to the assessment or collection of evidence are inappropriate. Questions that imply criticism of the victim are to be avoided. Examples of such questions are "Why aren't you crying?" or "Did you put up a fight?" or "What were you doing out at that time of night?" These are accurately perceived by the victim as judgmental and provocative.

Being *angry* with the victim for "getting herself raped" is a common emotion of many nurses. This is a defensive response to feelings of vulnerability. Every victim is a reminder that we too could be raped, a very threatening thought! The nurse needs to recognize this anger and understand that it serves the purpose of making her feel more secure and safe from the possibility of a similar fate. If she can find a way to see the victim as responsible for having been raped, then she can avoid being raped by never behaving that way.

Anger at the rapist is also common. It is important that the nurse not act on this feeling and coerce the victim into reporting the crime. That would be meeting the needs of the angry nurse rather than the victim.

Notifying the police is always the victim's decision. The nurse can support the victim as she struggles with the decision but should not force her opinion on the victim. It would also be totally unacceptable for the nurse to notify the police without the victim's consent. The victim, not the nurse, must live with the situation once the police are involved.

If the victim elects to involve the police, the nurse will provide support throughout the police interviews when they occur in the EU. At that time, the nurse may find herself responding angrily to law enforcement personnel if they are not sensitive or skilled in dealing with the victim. In this case, she needs to try to aid the officer by rephrasing his questions or directing him to understand the victim's sensitivity.

Other areas also present themselves as convenient targets for the nurse's anger: the parents of young victims, the male mates of older victims, the gynecologist, or the assigned counselor, especially if the latter is not available to be with the victim and thus leaves the nurse to deal with a situation in which she may feel uncomfortable or inadequate. If need be, the nurse should be prepared to deal competently with the victim alone. The nurse must be aware of her own feelings so that she does not inappropriately express them in relation to the victim, to the victim's family members, or to teammates.

A particularly difficult situation that can provoke anger in the nurse is the patient who refuses care or refuses to go along with hospital protocol. This situation is provocative because the victim, by asserting herself, has shifted control away from the nurse to herself. Loss of control is threatening to anyone, especially to nurses geared to taking charge and doing what needs to be done.

The nurse must realize that this refusal is not a personal affront nor ingratitude; rather, it is the victim's legitimate prerogative and personal response to a difficult situation. Understanding this, the nurse will find that she does not need to respond angrily in return. An example of such a situation was related by an EU nurse from a hospital that sees many victims:

> This unaccompanied woman came in and said she wanted to be treated for VD because she was just raped. I immediately began to call people on the protocol and told her the rape counselor would be right down. Well, she said she wouldn't talk with him! She didn't want to talk with him or me or the police or anybody. She only wanted a penicillin shot. I was furious with her, but she couldn't be reasoned with, and then I realized I was being ridiculous and antagonizing her more. I then agreed to treat her for exposure to VD, and before she left, she even let me give her the rape counseling phone number.

In a case like this, the nurse, by hearing the victim's request, establishes a good rapport with her. Then the victim, who is not immediately amenable to the idea of counseling, will understand that the door is always open.

In particularly difficult cases, the nurse may also find that she responds angrily because she is frustrated in her efforts to care for the victim with special needs. One nurse said,

> A mother brought in her severely retarded daughter who had been raped. The mother was very supportive with her but also very protective, maybe overprotective. Because the girl was badly hurt, we felt we had to do the physical exam immediately. I felt so helpless. Nobody could make the girl understand but the mother, and the mother was so upset she could hardly talk to me, let alone to the girl. She was terrified when we put her in the stirrups, and only keeping the mother there seemed to help.

One will often find in this type of case that both mother and daughter require supportive counseling. While the victim is being examined may be a good opportunity for the mother or family members to vent their feelings to the counselor. The need for this type of intervention will often be identified by the nurse, who can then share the information with the counselor when planning the care.

Occasionally, the nurse will discover that she is acting out her angry feelings inappropriately, that is, that she is displacing her anger onto the victim. An example is given by a nurse at a suburban hospital that infrequently treats rape victims:

> It was 2:30 P.M. when the police brought her in. It was my turn to take the next victim, and, of course, one *would* come the day I was supposed to pick up a friend at the airport after work. At our EU, you stay with the victim as long as they're in. It's usually several hours. I was fuming around the place and overheard the victim's friend ask the policewoman if we were always so nasty with rape victims at this hospital. I realized it was me they were talking about. I felt rotten. It wasn't her fault she got raped. I called my husband to go to the airport, and then I apologized to her. Then I tried to make it up to her. It was 5 P.M. before I got out of there, but everybody understood when I finally got home.

In the above situation, the nurse was responding with anger to a reality issue, that of the interruption of her plans, not to dealing with a rape victim.

Doubt or skepticism in relationship to a victim can be extremely difficult for both victim and nurse. Resulting from either the victim's story or the manner of presentation, doubt can interfere with the provision of good care if the nurse is not able to control her verbalization or behavior. Despite these feelings, the victim is entitled to every aspect of good care recommended in the protocol. Rapes sometimes occur under bizarre circumstances, and all victims respond in their own personality style (Williams & Williams, 1973). An example:

> This woman came in at 3 A.M. She was absolutely filthy, and the odor of booze was so strong it could knock you down. Then she said she had been raped at the parking lot of a local bar. Well, I was so disgusted by her appearance and behavior that I wanted to avoid her but couldn't because I was the only nurse on. I could hardly believe her story, but in her condition, she certainly was vulnerable. We implemented the protocol and on exam found several vaginal tears and severe contusions. I felt terrible for not having believed her immediately. I only hope my skepticism didn't show through.

When the story seems implausible or there is no evidence of sperm or semen on exam or the victim does not behave in an expected manner, it does not mean that rape has not occurred. The nurse who is subjectively doubtful should be very careful to remain objective and not share these reservations with family or police. The risk is that the nurse's personal opinion could be misconstrued as a professional opinion. The relationship between the victim and either of these groups has the potential to be difficult in the most clearcut of cases. Complicating these relationships by mention of any opinion can be destructive, unfair, and certainly at odds with the victim's best interests, especially if court proceedings are a possibility.

Hospital and Community Issues

Hospital and community issues are important considerations in providing a victim with good nursing care. Recognizing the special needs of rape victims has yielded a variety of methods for dealing with this emergency. When possible, the multidisciplinary team approach is employed to manage all aspects of victim care. It has long been witnessed in the actual provision of health care that the ideal is not always available and that the nurse is the one to whom the multiple tasks fall. This fact dictates that nurses be flexible and prepared in order to provide the best possible care for the victim. With that in mind, the nurse may find that she is not only a member of the "rape crisis team" but may be the coordinator of the team. In hospitals with a small incidence of rape victims, where a formal team is not felt to be needed, she may be "the rape person." When this occurs, the nurse must adapt recommendations whenever possible to her particular hospital system.

The nurse who is the key person for coordinating the EU care of rape victims will find that there are certain stresses that go with the job. Within the hospital system, some stresses may come from the hospital administration. While generally supportive of the idea, they are also concerned because their public image is at stake. In the case of hospitals with strong religious beliefs, there may be conflict over the use of postcoital contraception or referral for menstrual extraction or therapeutic abortion. These are very difficult and delicate areas to be negotiated. The nurse, in her historic role as patient advocate, must work with hospital authorities to assure the provision of information and services to victims without compromising hospital ethics.

Nursing service administration needs to support the provision of this specialized care. This support is demonstrated by allowing the nursing coordinator freedom to spend time researching what is available in the local or regional community. She will need to determine what is needed, to establish liaisons, and to have ongoing meetings with necessary groups in and out of the hospital. Support then needs to be broadened to include educational preparation of the nursing coordinator via appropriate courses or workshops dealing with the rape trauma syndrome, crisis intervention theory, etc. The need for ongoing meetings and in-service training to sensitize, educate, and deal with feelings evoked in all EU personnel is another form the support must take (Brodyaga et al., 1975). Provision also needs to be made for the occasion when a nurse will need to work beyond regularly scheduled shifts in order to remain with the victim in the EU.

Nursing coordinators, especially of new or infrequently utilized programs, need ongoing meetings with those in similar positions at other institutions. Sharing information on resources, new research findings, protocol recommendations, etc., will aid the coordinator in maintaining her efficiency, interest, and concern. Through peer support and supervision, these discussions will stimulate creative thinking and lead to problem anticipation, identification, prevention, and solution.

On a smaller scale, the nursing coordinator may find that the pressure from her co-workers will take an unusual form. Some will provide wholehearted support; others will want absolutely nothing to do with the proposed program and may be openly disgusted or angry at the idea of being asked to take part. Co-workers may assume that the interested nurse has been a rape victim herself at one time. This fantasy will be more prevalent among groups of people who have not been sensitized to rape. How the nurse chooses to deal with this fantasy will depend on her personal style. Open discussion of the fact versus the fantasy is the ideal method for curtailing this belief.

Because of the sensational nature of rape, the nurse who works with victims will find that some co-workers pressure her to tell what she knows of the gory details. This morbid curiosity and the nurse's need to ventilate her feelings about anxiety-provoking cases may combine to make her vulnerable to an unintentional breach of confidentiality. To avoid this risk, the nurse needs to have an appropriate place to discuss the case and to gain some distance from it as well as to get help with her feelings. Providing oneself with an appropriate place to talk can greatly decrease the possibility of inappropriate spilling of information.

Within the hospital, the nurse must negotiate with the pharmacy in order to have them stock whatever postcoital contraception will be provided via the protocol. The laboratory will need to cooperate in having microscope facilities available in either the lab or the EU, for the examining gynecologist to use in checking slides for sperm. A system needs to be developed whereby the results of lab work can be given to the rape team nurse in order for her to refer the victim appropriately after the emergency aspect of her case is over. When the hospital has outpatient gynecology and VD clinics, liaison must be made with them to smooth the way for the victim, should a return checkup be indicated. The rape team nurse should be available to consult with the clinics for protocol development for their individual departments.

The relationship between the gynecologist and the nurse needs to be kept in good working order. Large hospitals with gynecological teaching programs will have a gynecology resident on call at the hospital and thus readily available to care for victims. These on-the-premises physicians are relatively accessible for the purpose of education about the protocol and sensitization to the needs of victims. In small community hospitals without gynecological teaching services, coverage is usually provided by a rotating on-call list of gynecologists in private practice. This group as a whole are more difficult to reach for the educative purposes. Where victims rarely present to the EU, the physician will probably not be immediately familiar with the protocol. In these instances, the nurse must be able to provide him with the protocol for his perusal before the exam begins. It is important at times like this that the nurse act as patient advocate to assist the physician in providing complete care, especially with regard to the use of postcoital contraception and VD prophylaxis.

On these occasions, the physician may experience many of the same emotions the nurse has experienced. The sophisticated nurse will understand this process and will be able to respond to his anxiety with reassurance and support rather than annoyance or anger. The victim will be sensitive to the physician's mood and may respond with anger or increased fear and anxiety. The nurse can reassure her that the gynecological exam is routine and that the physician has performed it numerous times.

Liaison with community agencies will facilitate the victim's ability to move from one to another with a minimum of trauma. Whenever possible, the nurse should give the victim the name of a key person to make the transition smooth. Liaison with the local law enforcement agency will increase its referral of victims for emergency care and will give the nurse an opportunity to identify which officers are truly sensitive and responsive. The nurse will then be able to confidently refer victims who have been uncertain about reporting for fear of how they will be treated. This particular liaison is also useful in providing the feedback necessary for evaluation of the emergency service.

Another useful aspect of this liaison with the law enforcement agency is that the nurse, with the victim's consent, can alert the police to the presence of a rapist in the vicinity by using the "anonymous report." Since it is a fact that most rapists rape more than once, this information along with facts about the modus operandi would be especially useful in apprehending the rapist. The "anonymous report" is an informal communication between the nurse and the police. The victim need never talk with police. The nurse assumes this task. Victims will not be identified to the police and can tell the nurse exactly what details can be shared. An example of a third-party (anonymous) report can be found in Appendix 4.

Other community agencies that need to be worked with are the community mental health center that will provide follow-up counseling when the hospital does not offer such services. A special item to be worked out is the need for victims to be seen quickly. Also, they should not be passed from intake worker to assigned counselor; instead, they should be seen immediately by the person who is going to work with them. This procedure eliminates the need for the victim to tell her story repeatedly.

Emergency units of hospitals that do not provide menstrual extraction or therapeutic abortion need to develop a liaison with a community agency that will meet this need.

Some communities have volunteer groups that work with the victim who decides to go through the legal process. If such a group is available, the victim should have the benefit of its expertise as soon as possible after the rape in order to prepare herself for the legal process. This service should be explained by the nurse, who can give the victim the name and numbers to call.

Community agencies for battered women and refuges where they can spend the night safely when afraid of returning home would be valuable resources for the nurse to share with victims.

In conclusion, via primary nursing the victim is offered a relationship in which she can plan for care according to her wants and needs. The primary nurse is accountable to the victim for that care.

Emergency nursing care of rape victims is complex. Preparation of staff and ongoing meetings are necessary to achieve and maintain sensitivity to rape as well as to help staff deal appropriately with the emotions evoked. Ongoing program evaluation is a major component in providing appropriate nursing care to these victims.

Effective collaboration facilitates the entire process, giving the victim access to crisis intervention and medical–gynecological treatment. Follow-up is designed according to what the victim wishes, and the primary nurse remains an available resource after she leaves the emergency unit. The benefits to the victim are obvious. The benefit to the nurse is the knowledge that the victim has begun to regain control over her life because of meaningful support, comfort, and a minimum of further trauma. Satisfaction comes from having seen a difficult case through from beginning to end.

References

Appell, L., Baskin, D., & Smith, J. The first half hour. *The Journal of Practical Nursing,* 1976, *26*(1), 15–18, 34–35.

Bellack, J. P., & Woodard, P. B. Improving emergency care for rape victims. *Journal of Emergency Nursing,* 1977, *5–6,* 32–35.

Brodyaga, L., Gates, M., Singer, S., Tucker, M., & White, R. *A report for citizens, health facilities, and criminal justice agencies.* Washington, D.C.: National Institute of Law Enforcement and Criminal Justice Law Enforcement Assistance Administration, U.S. Department of Justice, 11, 1975, pp. 75–80.

Burgess, A. W., & Holmstrom, L. L. The rape victim in the emergency ward. *American Journal of Nursing,* 1973, *10,* 1741–1745.

Hilberman, E. *The rape victim.* Washington, D.C.: American Psychiatric Association, 1976, pp. 22–28.

Klingbeil, K. S., Anderson, S. C., & Vontver, L. Multidisciplinary care for sexual assault victims. *Nurse Practitioner,* 1976, *7–8,* 21–25.

Little, D. E., & Carnevali, D. L. *Nursing care planning.* Philadelphia, Pa.: J. B. Lippencott, 1976, pp. 179–194.

Logsdon, A. Why primary nursing? *Nursing Clinics of North America,* 1973, *6*(2), 283–291.
Manthey, M., Ciske, K., Robertson, P., & Harris, I. Primary nursing. *Nursing Forum,* 1970, *9*(1), 65–83.
Williams, C. C., & Williams, R. A. Rape: A plea for help in the emergency room. *Nursing Forum,* 1973, *12*(4), 388–401.

5

The Medical Examination
Treatment and Evidence Collection

HENRY KLAPHOLZ

Fear of the hospital has kept many rape victims from seeking appropriate and timely medical attention. To some women, the gynecological examination can seem like a reenactment of the rape itself. As one rape victim put it, "The pelvic examination was quite depressing at the time. To have to get undressed again and get up on that table and go through almost the same thing again of something being stuck into you was awful." A proper, thoughtful, well-explained examination is essential if the gynecologist is to deliver good medical care to the victim, and good medical care should be his first priority.

His second priority should be to provide medical substantiation for the victim's story in case she should go to court. Although the gynecologist should record no conclusion about whether or not he thinks a rape actually occurred, he can do much to document his observations of signs of penetration, ejaculation, and abnormal force. By means of laboratory tests, physical findings, and the history he takes, his comments in the medical record add considerable weight in court to the victim's story.

A gynecological examination is not mandatory after a rape. No one may force a woman to be examined, and if the examination is refused, it is best simply to explain the procedure and the benefits that accrue from its performance. One should not press the issue further. Her refusal does not preclude treatment for venereal disease or possible pregnancy. It has been my experience that after proper counseling and explanation, most women

HENRY KLAPHOLZ, M.D. ● Assistant Professor of Obstetrics and Gynecology, Harvard Medical School; Coordinator of Medical Education, Department of Obstetrics and Gynecology, Beth Israel Hospital, Boston, Massachusetts.

are willing, and in fact desire, to be examined both for their physical well-being and for medical evidence.

A medical guideline for the gynecological care of a rape victim can be found in Appendix 2 of this book. Here, I will outline the basic aspects of the history taking, examination, and treatment of a rape victim, explaining the reasons behind the procedures whenever possible.

A complete and careful medical history should be taken. Drug allergies and other preexisting conditions affecting any therapy should be noted. Coagulation defects, hypertension, migraine, seizure disorders, and other matters pertaining to any treatments recommended must be noted in order to prevent serious medical and legal problems. It is bad medical practice for a gynecologist to prescribe antibiotic or hormonal therapy without such important information.

In planning any treatment program for the victim, contraceptive information is essential. If a reliable method of contraception has been used, such as the birth control pill or an intrauterine device (IUD), then the risk of pregnancy is small, and I do not usually recommend any further steps aimed at pregnancy prevention. Even if the assailant used a condom (and some do), this seems to me inadequate to prevent pregnancy with a high degree of certainty, and I would recommend further treatment. If the victim is sexually active, the possibility of a preexisting pregnancy must be considered; if it is a desired pregnancy, postcoital contraception would endanger the desired pregnancy.

The circumstances of the attack must be reviewed for two reasons. First, it will help the physician to direct his medical questioning more appropriately. Second, the recording of the history on the medical record will reinforce the legal evidence that the victim may later need. A physician's report of the victim's story is not, however, a requisite in all states; sometimes, the physician is called upon only to offer statements regarding the victim's emotional and physical state at the time of the examination. In any event, the gynecologist should remember that he is not a law enforcement officer; neither is he a judge or jury. The manner in which he takes the medical history should not seem legalistic or accusatory.

In the interest of proper medical treatment and substantiation of the victim's story in court, the gynecologist should be sure to ask about the following circumstances. Unusual sexual acts such as anal or oral intercourse should be noted. The geographic location of the assault—for example, on sandy ground, in a clay-filled area, on concrete, or on a wooden floor —can guide the physician to look for evidence of sand, clay, abrasions, or wooden splinters during his physical exam. Assault with any solid objects and blows to parts of the body other than the genital organs must likewise be asked about and confirmed by examination. Penetration and ejaculation (in the vagina or outside of it) should be asked about, as well. The number of assailants and their coloring should be noted, because pubic hair taken from the victim will often reveal hairs from the assailant(s) that may be helpful in the victim's formal identification of the rapist(s) for the trial.

Unfortunately, in many states, the issue of prior sexual experience is permitted to be used by defense attorneys in an attempt to make the woman appear promiscuous. Any sexual history taken by the gynecologist should be written in the record with this in mind. Only sexual history pertinent to present and future medical treatment should be included. A small, tight introitus, on the other hand, could materially aid a rape victim as corroboration of no previous sexual activity. It is well to remember that when the victim comes to court, the assailant's defense attorney often will ask questions in this regard, even if the physician has written nothing about contraception or intercourse in the record.

I routinely also ask about the use of cleansing douches or tampons following the rape. Many women feel dirty following the attack and will attempt to wash out the semen with a douche prior to appearing for examination and in the process will destroy evidence of semen or sperm in the vagina. The use of either tampon or douche should be recorded in the chart.

Even a woman who agrees to be examined can be somewhat ambivalent about it and very emotionally sensitive. Also, a good examination is impossible without the cooperation of the woman. For these reasons, it is necessary that the gynecologist be sensitive to her feelings and that he explain what he is doing. Acknowledgment of the woman's feelings in statements like "I know this is difficult" can do much good. It is normal for people working with rape victims to feel uncomfortable and under stress, but it is important that these feelings not preclude good medical care. Acknowledging these sensitive issues to oneself and to the victim can help to minimize the possibility of their obstructing the patient's medical–legal needs.

The physical examination must be painstakingly thorough, and all pertinent findings should be noted. If the history has been taken in adequate detail, this task is simplified considerably, since the physician will be guided by the story he has heard. The patient's general overall appearance should be noted and her mental state assessed. The state of her clothing and underclothing should also be noted as well as any change of clothes. If the patient has changed, it is wise to have her bring her old clothes in and store them in a bag as evidence for the police. If this is not feasible, the woman should be instructed to preserve the clothing herself.

Physical trauma, such as bruises, cuts, and scratches, should be noted with respect to location and apparent age. An estimated 50% of raped women show signs of physical trauma, most commonly on the face, arms, head, legs, and throat (Burgess & Holmstrom, 1973). Bruises to the body are usually from fists, and abrasions of the back and legs are frequently seen as the result of a struggle on the ground. The breasts as well as the genitals should be examined for evidence of trauma. It has been estimated that 5–8% of rape victims undergo genital trauma during the attack, and the hymen is the most frequently injured structure, followed by the vagina and the perineum (Burgess & Holmstrom, 1973). I have seen severe injuries to the vaginal wall resulting in massive hemorrhage from intercourse alone in an unprepared woman. It is equally important to examine the fornices (depths of the vagina) to determine if any serious trauma has occurred. There are cases of broomsticks, bottles, and other large or sharp foreign objects being forced up the vagina and into the abdominal cavity. Such injuries are life-threatening and must be dealt with immediately.

A bimanual examination will help to determine if any preexisting pregnancy is present. This portion of the examination must sometimes be omitted if the emotional state of the patient does not permit it. In such cases, the laboratory must be used to detect a pregnancy.

Pertinent laboratory studies must be done to ensure that the patient has not been innoculated with either gonorrhea or syphilis. A cervical culture for gonorrhea should be taken when the patient is first seen, prior to any treatment. Cultures of the rectum and the pharynx are appropriate if the history includes intercourse by these routes. A serological test for syphilis should be obtained as a baseline. Most authors on the subject agree that an immediate serology is useful as a starting point for comparison of later serologies (Hayman, 1975). A repeat serology four weeks after the rape will document that exposure has occurred if it is positive and the baseline negative.

Fluid should be aspirated from the posterior fornix of the vagina and sent to the laboratory for analysis for acid phosphatase (an enzyme found in high concentration in human semen) (Enos, Beyer, & Mann, 1972). A wet preparation of the vaginal secretions should be examined on the spot by the gynecologist to determine the presence of active, motile sperm. Sperm can remain viable for several days but are rarely viable after 12 hours. This examination must be done in the emergency room and cannot be sent to a laboratory, for the slide will dry out and the sperm die. The results of the wet preparation should be noted in the record. In addition, a Papanicolaou type of preparation of the vaginal secretions should be sent to the laboratory to confirm the finding of sperm. Bear in mind that none of these tests establishes a rape. They merely confirm that at some time, somehow, sperm and/or semen were introduced into the vagina. There is no definitive means at hand to determine the owner or the route of administration.

Smears of suspicious areas on the vulva or other areas reported to have been ejaculated upon should be sent at well. Then, foreign pubic hairs should be collected and sealed for examination by the police laboratory if the patient wishes. Such evidence may be useful in identifying or ruling out an alleged assailant at the trial.

It is estimated that 1 in 20 women subjected to undesired intercourse get some form of venereal disease, usually gonorrhea (Hayman, Lanza, & Fuentes, 1969). One need not, however, diagnose the existence of venereal disease in order to prescribe treatment, although considerable disagreement exists in the medical community as to whether diagnosis must precede treatment. In my opinion, every rape victim should be given the benefit of prophylactic antibiotic therapy.

For gonorrhea, provided the patient is not allergic to penicillin, the present recommended treatment is 4.8 million units of penicillin accompanied by an oral dose of Probenecid. If the patient is allergic to penicillin, one gives spectinomycin (2 grams) as an injection. In contrast to the treatment of most infectious diseases, we do not wait for cultures to confirm exposure, because 5–10% of cultures may be falsely negative, and a delay in treatment may be disastrous to the woman. Venereal disease may be transmitted to the pharynx and the rectum as well as to the genitals, and, therefore, one must inquire about these forms of sexual assault. Appropriate cultures from these sites should be obtained to document exposure to gonorrhea.

Serology for syphilis turns positive only three weeks after exposure. The prophylaxis for syphilis depends on the patient's allergies. If she has been given penicillin, she has already been protected against incubating syphilis and needs no further treatment. If she is allergic to penicillin and has received spectinomycin, she should be followed with serial blood tests for syphilis, since syphilis cannot be treated with spectinomycin.

Follow-up visits to a gynecologist are indicated to see if venereal warts (condylomata acuminata) have been transmitted. These can be treated easily while small and circumscribed. If left alone, they can reach huge dimensions and a major operation might be required to remove them. If herpes hominis type 2 (genital herpes) has been transmitted, the gynecologist can provide supportive treatment until the lesions subside. There is at present no prophylactic treatment against herpes or warts.

The grief of an unwanted pregnancy is compounded when the pregnancy is the result of rape. It is the duty of the gynecologist to offer whatever medical means are at his disposal to reduce the chance of pregnancy and to terminate any pregnancy that might arise as a result of the undesired intercourse.

The most commonly prescribed drug for the prevention of pregnancy had been diethylstilbestrol (DES). This drug possesses estrogenic properties and is believed to work by altering the Fallopian tube motility and rendering the lining of the uterus inhospitable to a fertilized ovum. The usual dose was 25 milligrams twice a day for five days. Other estrogens can be used; intravenous Premarin is often prescribed. The most common side effects of these medications are nausea and irregular vaginal bleeding. Antiemetics, such as Trilafon or Compazine, are frequently given along with estrogens to prevent the nausea and vomiting. These antinausea drugs are usually taken one-half to three-quarters of an hour prior to the estrogen.

Recent reports of abnormalities in the offspring of women who had been subjected to DES ingestion during pregnancy have raised some concern about the use of this and similar agents as postcoital contraceptives. Cancer of the vagina (a very rare disorder) and vaginal adenosis (a common but benign disorder) have both been found in offspring of mothers who ingested DES during pregnancy (Herbst, Ulfelder, & Poskanzer, 1971). Because of these findings, we no longer recommend this or similar drugs to the rape victim. If estrogens are taken in an attempt to prevent pregnancy, abortion should be offered if the treatment fails.

The question of coagulation defects and the increased risk of thromboembolic phenomena (specifically thrombotic strokes) in users of oral contraceptives has posed the same problem for the users of postcoital contraceptives containing estrogens. At present, we have no data that define the actual increased risk one incurs by taking DES, but it can be assumed to be small, since the medication is taken for only five days.

Another method of postcoital contraception that has recently been shown to be effective is the immediate insertion of an IUD. The mechanism of the IUD is obscure at present, but it is believed to prevent implantation of the fertilized ovum in the endometrial (uterine) cavity (Oldershaw, 1975). It is presumed that the IUD acts similarly when employed as a postcoital contraceptive.

We routinely advise all rape victims to have a pregnancy test performed five weeks after the rape in order to ensure that they are not pregnant. It is possible to bleed even while pregnant, thereby giving a false impression that the woman is having her menstrual period. A delay of four weeks increases the risk associated with abortion and may often change the type of abortion procedure required from a safe, simple one to a more complicated one. Some women, believing that they are immune from pregnancy by virtue of having taken DES, may also fail to seek medical attention even in the face of 10 or 12 weeks of amenorrhea (no periods). It is the duty of the gynecologist seeing the woman for the first time to inform her of these possibilities and to arrange for a follow-up examination and pregnancy test. A pregnancy test at the time the woman is initially seen should be performed, especially if postcoital contraception is to be prescribed, in case she was pregnant before the rape occurred.

The process of menstrual extraction or menstrual regulation has been adopted by some in order to avoid the wait for the positive pregnancy test. It also frees the victim from any guilt or shame she may associate with having become pregnant by a rapist, since by this method there is never any verification as to whether she actually was pregnant or not. Care must be taken with menstrual extractions performed at the time of exposure, since they have been known to miss the pregnancy, leaving the woman with a false sense of security.

If the victim returns to the office for follow-up and is found to be pregnant, she may be offered a simple vacuum curetage. This is a safe, rapid, inexpensive, and relatively comfortable procedure that is easily performed on her as a hospital outpatient under local or general anesthesia. There are freestanding abortion clinics in most parts of the country that provide these services at costs somewhat lower than hospital costs.

In addition to offering the aforementioned medical and legal protections, the gynecologist can initiate the emotional rehabilitation of the rape victim. Reassurance concerning her physical well-being is essential. A clear description of what the gynecologist has found, a clear course of action, and, most of all, understanding and sympathy must characterize his relationship with the patient. Her fears of death, pregnancy, and venereal disease must be handled with compassion and clarity. In this most trying of moments, it is often difficult for the physician to relate adequately to a sometimes hysterical, confused, injured, and, most of all, frightened individual. This is not the time to be authoritative, castigating, demeaning, jocular, informal, or curt. No time limit can be set on the emergency visit. Pressing medical needs take priority, of course, and sometimes speed in action must supplant a considered explanation, but barring such unusual circumstances, time must be given the victim to explain properly what is being done and why. Some rape interviews take only 10 minutes, others several hours. The physician must be able and willing to give whatever time is required without interruption.

House physicians, interns, and residents are often called on to evaluate a rape victim at late hours of the night, and they frequently respond to such calls with the reluctance one can expect of someone who has been working for 36 hours in a row and has just settled down to his first few hours of sleep. It takes only a few rape interviews, however, for one to realize that these patients require the same serious attention afforded the seriously wounded. They have, in fact, been wounded, not only physically but mentally as well. It is not good medical practice to let such patients undergo the stress of a long wait in the emergency room while a gynecologist is located. There is no legal requirement that the woman be examined by a gynecologist *per se*. With adequate training of emergency room personnel and the posting of the American College of Obstetrics and Gynecology Standards for Rape, the emergency room physician present can treat her and collect the proper specimens.

If available, a rape crisis intervention counselor can help the physician in understanding and dealing with the feelings of rape victims. If no such counselor is available, psychiatric consultation and follow-up care for the victim should be sought. Serious psychiatric sequelae that are not immediately obvious may surface days, or even months, after the actual occurrence of the rape.

In summary, the medical treatment of a rape victim is intended to deal with the physical and emotional needs of an injured woman at a time when she has been under acute stress. It is also a delicate but comprehensive search for medical evidence in support of the victim's assertion that she has had undesired, forced intercourse. The gynecological examination need never seem like "almost the same thing again" as the rape. Instead, it can do much to restore and reassure her about her health and, indeed, her faith in the compassion and understanding of other people.

References

Burgess, A. W., & Holmstrom, L. L. The rape victim in the emergency ward. *American Journal of Nursing*, 1973, *73*, 1741–1745.

Enos, W. F., Beyer, J. C., & Mann, G. T. The medical examination of cases of rape. *Journal of the Forensic Science Society*, 1972, *17*, 50–56.

Hayman, C. R. Guidelines for the interview and evaluation of the alleged rape victim. *Western Journal of Medicine*, 1975, *123*, 420–422.

Hayman, C. R., Lanza, C., & Fuentes, R. Sexual assault on women and girls in the District of Columbia. *Southern Medical Journal*, 1969, *62*, 1227–1231.

Herbst, A. L., Ulfelder, H., & Poskanzer, D. C. Adenocarcinoma of the vagina: Association of maternal stillbestrol treatment with tumor appearance in young women. *New England Journal of Medicine*, 1971, *22*, 878–881.

Oldershaw, K. L. *Contraception, sterilization and abortion.* New York: Year Book Medical Publishing, 1975.

III

The Legal System

Despite the fact that the rate of reported rape has increased by over 100% during the period from 1965 through 1974, the crime of rape remains one of the most underreported of the serious felonies. Empirical data are inconclusive regarding the reasons that victims of sexual assault decide not to report the incident to the authorities. The experience of counselors, police, and prosecutors working with victims indicates that the single most common reason for nonreporting is the victim's fear and uncertainty about her treatment in the legal system. One nationwide survey found that 53% of those victims who withdrew their rape complaints after having reported them to the police did so because of fear and embarrassment.[1] In our public education efforts, we have all too often heard women state that they would never report a rape to the police or testify in court because they expect this experience to be as harrowing as the assault itself.

In the immediate aftermath of the rape, the decision whether or not to report it to the police comes at a time when rational and reflective thought is most difficult. Compounding this dilemma is the victim's lack of information about the law and the criminal justice process. Unfortunately, the longer the victim delays in going to the police, the more her credibility is diminished and the less likely it is that a jury will find her assailant guilty.

It is important for hospital personnel and rape counselors to be familiar with both police and courtroom procedures in order to provide the victim with the information necessary for her to make her decision. This section is designed to give non-criminal-justice personnel a thorough understanding of what the victim can expect once she reports the rape to the police. It presents guidelines for law enforcement officers and prosecutors, detailing the methods and approaches that have proved most effective in securing the cooperation of victims as complaining witnesses. These chapters are not intended, however, to be a complete discussion of either the relevant law or the criminal justice process, since each state has its own statutes and cus-

[1]National Institute of Law Enforcement and Criminal Justice, *Forcible Rape: Police Volume I,* March 1977, p. 9.

toms. Readers are urged to research the specific law and procedures in their own jurisdictions. These chapters do make reference to recent reforms in rape statutes and changes in both police and prosecutor practices that may serve as models for other communities.

The chapter by Peter J. Murphy describes the stages in the police investigation, from the receipt of the call by the police clerk to the presentation of evidence in the courtroom. Murphy presents a model for investigation that stresses the importance of sensitivity to the victim. Concern for the victim is advocated not only for humane reasons but also to elicit her full cooperation in the investigation and prosecution. He argues for active liaison between the hospital, the district attorney's office, the rape counselor, and the police.

Alice E. Richmond's first chapter presents an overview of the evolution of laws regarding rape and an explanation of the criminal justice process. Most of us outside the police and legal professions are ignorant about the workings of the system. The experience of testifying in a criminal trial is difficult under any circumstances and is especially discomforting for the rape victim. It can be made less overwhelming if the victim understands what is happening and is properly prepared for it. Richmond contends that thorough, clearly detailed preparation is the key to making the victim a more comfortable and more effective witness. Her second chapter describes the various roles of all participants in the courtroom. It covers what is expected of the victim as her case moves toward trial and includes some suggestions about how to minimize her apprehension throughout the process.

6

The Police Investigation

PETER J. MURPHY III

Rape is second only to murder as the most serious crime a police officer faces. The responsibility of the police in a rape case is twofold: first, to protect and support the victim, with the ultimate goal of facilitating her complete psychological recovery; second, to apprehend and successfully prosecute the culprit. These are complementary objectives. Rape is one of the few crimes that require the full cooperation of the victim to bring about a successful prosecution.

In spite of the seriousness of the crime, many police officers in the past treated the victim in a way that was unprofessional. Unless the victim sustained obvious physical injury, many officers felt that the victim was probably "looking for it" and regarded the report as unfounded. This attitude was supported by the Massachusetts State statute that defined rape as "whoever ravishes and carnally knows a female *by force* and against her will."[1] Threats of violence were not considered use of force. The victim could sense that she was not believed by the police, and her cooperation with them would diminish or disappear.

In order to develop a bond of trust, the officer must be sympathetic and must be prepared to invest a lot of time in the investigation. The victim who is given the time to get herself back together after the initial trauma and to get to know the investigating officers will feel that the officers are really interested in her well-being and will be likely to continue the legal process.

In 1974, the Massachusetts Legislature passed two major pieces of legislation concerning rape. The first piece amended Chapter 265, Section 22, of the General Laws by redefining the criminal act of rape as "whoever

[1]Massachusetts General Laws Annotated. Chapter 265, Section 22.

PETER J. MURPHY III ● Detective, Brookline Police Department, Brookline, Massachusetts.

has sexual intercourse or unnatural sexual intercourse with a person, and compels such person to submit by threat of bodily injury, shall be punished by imprisonment in the state prison for life or for any term of years."[2] This legislation involved three major changes in the statute that should help both the victims and the police. The first is that force no longer has to be proved; the threat of bodily injury is sufficient. The second change is that unnatural sexual intercourse is now included in the statute. Before this change, the culprit who forced a victim to submit to unnatural intercourse (anal or oral intercourse) was charged with unnatural acts, a lesser crime, or possibly assault with intent to rape. The third change is that the law now recognizes that the victim may be male as well as female.

The second piece of legislation passed in 1974 is also of major significance. The Rottenberg Bill forced reform within the police departments of every city and town in the commonwealth.[3] The most important part of the bill requires that each department establish a rape reporting and prosecution unit. The units must be staffed by officers who have completed an approved course of training in the counseling of victims and the prosecution of the perpetrators. A second point of the bill is that each rape reporting and prosecution unit must establish a special telephone exchange for the reporting of rape. Third, the bill requires that all reports of rape, sexual assault, or attempts to commit those crimes and all conversations between police officers and victims shall not be public reports and shall be maintained in a manner that will assure their confidentiality.

Since the Rottenberg Bill was made law, the Massachusetts Criminal Justice Training Council has been training officers throughout the commonwealth to staff the units. The objectives are better treatment of rape victims and more successful prosecutions. These reform measures may be taken as models for other states working to improve the police investigation of rape cases.

The police who respond to the rape call consist of three groups: the police clerk, the patrol unit, and the detective unit. Each has a sequential role in the protection of the victim and in the apprehension and prosecution of the rapist.

When a victim calls the police to report that she has been raped, the clerk is generally the first person to whom she speaks. It is the duty of the clerk to determine if the call is an emergency (almost all are). A rape that has just occurred, one where the victim is injured, or one where the victim is in obvious emotional distress is classified as an emergency. This type of call requires an immediate response by the patrol division. Complaints that are delayed several days after the rape may be investigated entirely by the

[2]Ibid.
[3]Massachusetts General Laws Annotated. Chapter 581, 1974.

specialized rape unit. The clerk taking the call should determine what the victim's name is, where she is calling from, where the attack occurred, when it occurred, the culprit's description, and the direction and means of flight. A patrol car and the rape unit (if immediately available) are dispatched directly to aid the victim. The clerk should try to keep the victim on the telephone until the officers arrive. This communication gives the victim a feeling of safety and ensures that the victim will be in the location from which she called. This time on the telephone may be used to get a better description of the attacker but not to pry into the details of the attack.

The patrol officer is almost always the first officer to arrive at the scene. He should identify himself to the victim. The officer's first task is to assess the victim's physical condition and to express concern for her well-being. The victim's trust may be gained simply by showing an interest in how she is. One officer should interview the victim briefly to determine what happened, where, when, and by whom. If the identity of the culprit is unknown, a description must be obtained to assist the other units in their search for him. This is only a brief interview and should not go into an indepth account of what happened. Unnecessary patrol units should not be permitted to congregate at the scene. The officer should take notes on the victim's physical and emotional condition for possible use in court later. The crime scene should be protected so that valuable physical evidence will not be lost. If the detectives assigned to the rape investigation unit are not available, the patrol officer should take the victim to the hospital. If necessary, the officer explains to the victim why a medical examination is important to her well-being. Ideally, hospital personnel are notified in advance so that those assigned to the rape crisis team will be prepared. This procedure eliminates undue delays in the treatment of the victim. If possible, the victim should bring an extra change of clothing to the hospital so that she can give her clothing to the police, because the clothing worn during the attack can provide investigators with many pieces of valuable physical evidence. Before leaving the hospital, the patrol officer should offer the victim transportation home and advise her that the rape investigators will be contacting her.

Each police department should have a rape investigation unit staffed by both male and female officers. Detectives should be assigned to this unit by virtue of their knowledge, experience, and sensitivity. Interviewing a rape victim can be one of the most challenging and sensitive duties a detective will ever have.

The police officer's response to rape victims may be influenced by his own response to crisis and to sexuality. The officer may hold the same misconceptions about rape as the general public. His personal style of responding to emergencies may lessen his effectiveness with rape victims. For example, the aggressive interrogation used in dealing with suspects can intimidate a victim and inhibit her full cooperation. Because the police officer functions in a male-dominated system, he may feel anxious and awkward when faced with a woman, particularly when his job calls for discussing sexual acts. Police are responsible for geographic sectors or beats. When a particularly serious crime occurs, the officer may feel that his territory has been violated or experience it as a personal failure. If an officer's attitude toward the victim is negative, it may well be the result of conflicts in his own emotional reaction to the event. In order to protect himself from feeling vulnerable, helpless, or anxious, he may unintentionally approach the case with the wish to believe that the crime is unfounded, thereby getting himself off the hook. Rape investigators, therefore, should be officers with the knowledge and experience to deal with their own feelings properly.

Although there is a difference of opinion on whether the investigating detective should conduct an in-depth interview immediately after the attack, this officer feels that the investigator should contact the victim as soon as possible but delay the detailed interview. Even though the patrol division can adequately handle the victim's immediate needs, a manifestation of interest in the victim during her time of acute crisis will help create a supportive and cooperative atmosphere between the victim and the investigator. Delaying the in-depth interview produces better victim cooperation, a more detailed account of what happened, and a more relaxed attitude on the victim's part. The investigator should advise the victim that he will be contacting her for a complete report when she is feeling better. In most cases, this should be the next day, but the timing depends on the victim's physical and emotional condition.

In the meantime, the investigation continues. As much physical evidence as possible is collected. The scene of the crime should be carefully examined. Pieces of torn clothing, signs of struggle or forced entry, objects dropped by the culprit, and fingerprints may be found. During the process of identifying a suspect, the detective selects from his collection of photographs of known sex offenders those men who fit the victim's description of the culprit. It is important not to arrange a photo lineup of too many subjects because a victim viewing too many photographs may have her memory of the subject's face distorted. The investigator sends a teletype message via computer to police departments throughout the state. The message includes the subject's physical description and his method of attack. If another police department has information that may identify the culprit, it transmits it to the department investigating the unsolved rape.

The rape investigator must determine exactly what happened and how it happened. An interview is arranged between the victim and the investigator. The in-depth interview should be conducted in a place with privacy, possibly the victim's home. A police station is a poor location for this interview. The victim is asked to tell what happened in her own words. She should be allowed to tell the story with no interruptions. After the victim has related the story, the investigator goes back over the story and asks questions. The investigator is trying to determine what type of personality he will be looking for, especially for a pattern linking this rapist with other reported rapes. To establish a suspect's modus operandi (MO), the investigator asks how the victim was first approached, what conversation transpired, what types of threats or violence were used, the sexual details, and how the culprit left. Statements and behavior of the culprit are very important.

A perfect example of how an MO can identify a rapist is illustrated by a recent case:

> A 37-year-old white female was grabbed from behind by a black male as she was entering her home. The culprit had a knife at the victim's throat and stated, "Don't move. I have a knife to your throat. Don't make a sound. You have a terrific body!" The victim was led to a bedroom and told to cover her eyes. The culprit then asked the victim a series of questions: "What's your name? Are you married? What's your age? When is your anniversary? Do you have sex?" The culprit then took pieces of tissue and put them in front of her eyes and tied them in place. The culprit told the victim that he would be her slave. He attempted to have intercourse with the victim but was unsuccessful. He then performed cunnilingus on the victim and told her that he would leave "after you come." The victim faked an orgasm. The culprit also told the victim that he wanted to take Polaroid pictures of her. Just before the culprit fled, he told the victim, "You've had such a good time you won't report me."

The detectives investigating this incident related the story to a detective in an adjacent town. The listener stopped the detectives midway through the report. He finished the story as though he were reading the report. He provided the name of a man arrested in his community who had used the same MO but who had not been convicted. The subject was arrested a month later during the commission of another rape and is now serving an 18- to 20-year sentence. At least 10 rapes have been solved by studying this subject's MO and providing the information to other investigators.

If the victim is willing, the interview should be tape-recorded so that an investigator will not have to repeatedly question a victim about a part of the attack that she may find difficult to speak about. The investigator must have patience and attempt to create an atmosphere that will allow the victim to deliver the necessary information willingly and naturally (Bard & Ellison, 1974). The manner and phrasing of questions is important. A good example of questioning is "It's not uncommon in this type of assault for a rapist to do things that are embarrassing to talk about . . . did anything like that happen to you?" The investigator should be prepared to answer any of the victim's questions. The victim may not understand why the investigator asks certain questions, particularly about the sexual aspects. The investigator should explain the importance of establishing a detailed MO and why he asks a particular question. In a later interview, the investigator should explain the court procedure to the victim. It is always important for the victim to know what to expect.

The police detective is the only person to follow the victim through each step of the legal process. An important task in this role is to maintain contact and support the victim so that she can function as an effective witness. Because of courtroom backlog and case continuances, it may take a year and a half to see the case to completion. This delay is demoralizing and stressful for the victim; she can become so discouraged that she drops the charges. By keeping the victim informed about the progress of the case, by educating her about the court system, and by supporting her resolve to testify, the detective can retain her as a witness. This process may entail daily contact in the initial stages and regular monthly telephone contact as the case progresses. The police officer prepares the victim for what to expect. For example, he warns her that private investigators hired by the defendant may contact her and try to appear official, but that she does not have to communicate with anyone but the police detective working with her on her case.

One rape victim required a great deal of personal contact with the investigator in the initial stages of the legal process. The victim had had a series of emotional setbacks in her life before the rape. The rape was a devastating experience for her. Besides having daily telephone counseling with her counselor, she wanted daily communication with the investigator. The victim developed a fear of the city in which the rape occurred and at first was unable to return to the city to meet with the detective. Three weeks after the attack, the victim was finally able to come and make a positive identification of the rapist. The rapist's identity was known to the investigator the day of the attack from information received from an informant, but because the victim was not ready, the identification procedure was delayed. The rapist was arrested. Three weeks later, probable cause was found in the municipal court. The investigator spoke with the victim almost daily during this three-week period. The victim was prepared and made an excellent witness.

One of the primary police responsibilities is the collection of evidence. All rape investigators deal with both people and things. When people commit rape, they almost always leave behind an assortment of things, such as fingerprints, hair, blood, semen, and clothing fibers, that make up what is known as *physical evidence.* It is important for the investigator to find it, properly collect it, and preserve it. These pieces of physical evidence are irrefutable and constitute the best type of evidence to present to the jury.

During a trial, juries have to decide whether or not the accused is guilty beyond a reasonable doubt. This decision can be most difficult. In a case where "consent" is the defense, it can be the seemingly insignificant piece of physical evidence collected by the police or the hospital personnel that will tip the balance. For example, a piece of torn bra strap recovered from the floor of the suspect's car or samples of skin and blood under the fingernails of the victim can be critical in corroborating use of force.

It is necessary to determine whether penetration—vaginal, oral, or anal—did occur and whether it was done by force or by threat of force. These are elements of the crime that must be proved in court. The collection of evidence may help to prove these elements. The rape investigator makes every attempt to obtain the clothing worn by the victim during the attack for laboratory examination. The garments should be examined for blood, semen, hair, clothing fibers, and other stains. The crime scene should be checked for evidence. In cases where the victim exhibits obvious physical injury, the police may ask the victim if they may photograph the injuries. The investigator must be sensitive to the fact that the victim has undergone a traumatic experience. By the time the case gets to court, the victim's physical wounds may have healed, but the photographs will show the victim as she looked after the attack. At the hospital, the victim is given a complete physical examination as well as a gynecological examination. All the victim's injuries should be noted on the medical report. The police are primarily interested in obtaining head and pubic hair combings, fingernail scrapings, and the results of the physical and gynecological examinations.

Physical evidence	What can be determined?
Hair	1. Whether the hair is human or animal in origin.
	2. The portion of the body from which the hair originated.
	3. Whether the hair was forcibly removed or fell out.
	4. Whether the person is Caucasian, Negroid, or Mongoloid.
	5. Whether the hair is similar to the hair of a person arrested.
Blood	1. Positive identification of human blood group A, AB, B, or O.
	2. Rh positive or Rh negative grouping.
	3. Whether blood does or does not contain rheumatoid arthritis factor.
	4. Presence of abnormal hemoglobins (sickle cells, etc.).
	5. Whether the stain is fetal, menstrual, or normal adult blood.
Semen	1. Positive identification of presence of semen.
	2. Positive A, B, O grouping of seminal fluid.
Clothing fiber	1. Whether the fiber could have come from a known source.
	2. Presence of blood or semen on fibers.
Fingernail scrapings	1. Skin samples or blood from assailant.

Rapes reported to the police are only a small fraction of the number of rapes that occur. The victim's decision on whether to report the rape is governed by many factors, which vary with each case. A victim may not call the police because of fear of the rapist; fear of the reaction of a husband, a boyfriend, or a parent; the desire to avoid further ordeal in the police and court process, etc. This decision can be made only by the victim. Yet, when the victim does not want to go to the police, valuable information may be lost. Police try to identify rapists through the information supplied by victims. Often, patterns develop. The identity of the rapist may be learned by putting together the information supplied by several victims. When cases go unreported, the rapist in a reported case may go unidentified or undetected because the police lack the necessary information.

One attempted solution to the problem of unreported cases is the use of a "third-party" rape report form, filled out by the victim at the hospital. The purpose of this form is to assist the police in identifying rapists when a victim does not want to go to the police. There is no effort on the part of the police to identify the victim when she wants to remain anonymous. This report gives the police a new source of information, namely, the silent victims. These forms are completed and sent directly to a designated member of the rape investigation unit. The police examine the data for patterns in their own community and contact other departments to see if the information will be of assistance to them. An arrest cannot be made on the basis of an anonymous report; however, the description may be useful in narrowing down suspects of rapes that are reported to the police. While the use of this form is new, the author is optimistic about its usefulness. An example of a third-party report form may be found in Appendix 4 to this book.

A major problem in prosecuting rape cases has been the long delay from the day the suspect is arrested to the day he goes to trial in superior court. This delay can often be a year or more. All the time the case is pending, the victim's normal routine may be upset. Many victims say, "I wish I could just forget the whole thing." One victim who suffered intensely during each court appearance and who longed for it to be over put the matter well. She said, "I want to start living again" (Burgess & Holmstrom, 1974). This long ordeal is something that victims of rape should not have to go through.

William Delahunt, Norfolk County District Attorney, has developed a violent crime project for Norfolk County in Massachusetts. The project may well become a model for other jurisdictions. The aim of the project is to bring the violent, the hardened, or the habitual offender to trial in the superior court within 90 days of the date of arrest. The project is designed to include all violent crimes, but we will look at the project only as it relates to rape.

Each district court is assigned an assistant district attorney who screens cases on a daily basis. After a review of the police report, a check of the defendant's record, and if possible an interview with police and civilian witnesses, the assistant decides if the case should be considered for the project. If the assistant determines that the case should be considered for the project, he confers about the case with the project director. It is the project director who decides whether or not to accept the case. Once a case is accepted for the project, it is assigned to an assistant district attorney, who immediately begins preparing the case. This assistant remains with the case until it is disposed of in the superior court. In the past, a victim could have two or more assistants working on the case. Under the new system, the victim does not have to go over everything every time there is a change of attorneys. Many of the cases go directly to the grand jury and bypass the probable-cause hearing. Even when a case requires a probable-cause hearing, it is expected that the matter can be handled within 90 days (Delahunt, 1976). The project is aimed at the criminal who must be taken off the street. The rapist certainly falls within this category. It is also hoped that by the speeding up of the process, the victim will recover from her ordeal sooner than she otherwise would.

Just as developing a good working relationship with the victim is imperative to the police objectives, so too is establishing close cooperation with hospital personnel.

Investigators and hospital personnel must learn and respect each other's needs. Hospital personnel are increasingly aware of the police requirements for a successful investigation and prosecution of the rapist. Likewise, the police now display more sensitivity toward the hospital personnel's objective of ensuring the full recovery of the victim. This education can be achieved by hospital participation in police in-service training programs and by police participation in the hospital's training of emergency unit and rape crisis personnel.

Improved communication results in concrete gains. Evidence collection, which is often a problem, can be handled in the emergency ward in a more professional manner through the use of a rape protocol to ensure that no part of the physical examination will go unrecorded in the victim's records.

Some victims who go to the hospital first are more likely to report the rape when they are given the names of officers who the hospital personnel know are sympathetic. Even if the victim does not decide to report the rape, the hospital can make a third-party rape report, helping the police gain valuable information from victims who for some personal reason do not want to go to the police. In addition, hospitals and police departments can work together effectively on programs designed to educate the public on how to prevent rape, what to do if raped, and what to expect consequently of the police and the hospital. If arrest and conviction rates in rape cases are to be improved, it is critical that the public be informed about community resources and the necessary steps in seeking care, preserving evidence, and entering the criminal justice system.

In this chapter, we have looked at the role of the police in assisting the victim and successfully apprehending and prosecuting the criminal. The police must cooperate closely with the district attorney and the hospital to perform both these tasks. It is the police who support the victim through the entire legal process and are responsible for collecting evidence, finding and arresting the accused, interviewing the arrested subject, reporting on the facts to the district attorney, and perhaps testifying in court. The objectives of the police are a speedy return to normal life for the victim and the just prosecution of the culprit.

References

Bard, M., & Ellison, K. Crisis intervention and investigation of forcible rape. *The Police Chief*, May 1974, 68–74.

Burgess, A. W., & Holmstrom, L. L. *Rape: Victims of Crisis.* Bowie, Md.: Robert J. Brady, 1974, pp. 202–204.

Delahunt, W. Violent crime project for Norfolk county guidelines. Memorandum to District Court Assistant District Attorneys, District Court Administrators, Police Prosecutors, Dedham, Mass., July 12, 1976.

7

Rape Law and the Judicial Process

ALICE E. RICHMOND

When we hear that someone has been raped, the commonsense understanding of that expression is that a person, usually a woman, has been forced to have intercourse. But what is the legal definition of *rape*? Are there different degrees of rape? What about sodomy, fellatio, cunnilingus? If a woman is forced to commit these acts, is that "rape" as well? What is indecent assault and battery? Does the age of the victim or the rapist make any difference? At law, can males be raped as well? In order to answer these questions, it is necessary to explain briefly the evolutionary process of Anglo-American law.

Historical Background of Rape Law

All conduct that we define as "criminal" may be divided into two categories. Those acts (e.g., parking in a tow-away zone) that are not intrinsically "wrong" but that are declared illegal by a legislative body are called *malum prohibitum*. Those acts (e.g., murder) that are deemed by society to be inherently evil are called *malum per se* or "evil in and of itself."[1]

In England, where our legal tradition began, conduct that was *malum per se* was considered criminal under the common law even before the Parliament passed any specific statute prohibiting it. Briefly stated, com-

---

[1]Malum per se is also known as *malum en se*. For a more detailed definition of these phrases, see H. C. Black, *Black's Law Dictionary* (rev. 4th ed.) (St. Paul, Minn.: West Publishing, 1968), pp. 445–446, 1112.

ALICE E. RICHMOND, ESQ. ● Former Assistant District Attorney, Suffolk District; former Assistant Professor, New England School of Law, Boston, Massachusetts.

mon law is that body of law that is "judge-made"; it embodies the "usages and customs of immemorial antiquity"[2] as interpreted by courts, as opposed to laws that have been enacted by a legislature, or statutory law.

As Parliament began enacting laws making certain conduct "criminal," it became necessary to differentiate between "serious" crimes, for which the penalty was death and loss of all possessions and property, and "not-so-serious" crimes, which had lesser penalties. Thus, the "serious" crimes became known as *felonies* and the "not-so-serious" crimes became *misdemeanors*. The distinction between the two was, and is, defined by the punishment imposed on the offender after conviction. For example, under federal criminal law, a crime that is punishable by more than one year in prison is a felony; all others are misdemeanors. In most states, crimes that provide that the convicted offender may be sentenced to a state prison or penitentiary for any term of years are generally felonies. Misdemeanors are crimes that carry no possibility of imprisonment or provide only for relatively limited detention in a house of correction or a county jail.

Since the act of rape was considered *malum per se,* it was a common-law crime even before Parliament passed any laws defining it as a crime. Both at common law and under statutory law, rape was considered a felony and the punishment was death. Before a defendant could be convicted, it was necessary to show that he had engaged in *"illicit carnal knowledge of a female by force and against her will."*[3] Thus, initially, rape was a crime that, by definition, could be committed only by a man against a woman.

Over time, each word in the definition came to have a specific meaning under law. To prove that the carnal knowledge was "illicit," it was necessary to show that the defendant and the victim were not married; the only legal intercourse between a man and woman occurred if they were married to each other. Any other intercourse was "illicit." It follows that under common law a husband was legally incapable of raping his wife since, by definition, intercourse between a husband and wife was not illicit. This distinction has survived to contemporary times, and, although some states have abolished the rigid rule that a husband cannot rape a wife, it is still a legal impossibility in most states. The sole exception to this rule is that a husband *who assists another man* in the rape of his wife may be charged with and convicted of rape.

The second phrase, "carnal knowledge," eventually became defined as sexual intercourse.[4] To prove rape at common law and in most American jurisdictions, there must be testimony or evidence that the male's penis

[2]Ibid., pp. 345–346.
[3]Ibid., p. 1427.
[4]*Commonwealth* v. *Piccerillo,* 256 Mass. 487,489 (1926); *Commonwealth* v. *Squires,* 97 Mass. 59, 61 (1867).

entered the female's vagina. The least amount of penetration is sufficient, and it is not legally necessary that the male ejaculate. However, in the absence of any testimony or evidence of penetration by the penis, the defendant may not be convicted of rape.

Traditionally, only a female could be raped and only a male could be charged with rape. Eventually, however, a woman who assisted a male in raping another woman could also be charged with rape.

The two phrases that provided the most discussion and controversy involved what constituted "force" and what intercourse was "against the female's will." Force was generally viewed as the "violent" penetration of the woman that caused the woman both "injury" and "outrage."[5] However, the woman was *not* required, even at common law, to resist the male to the "utmost" of her ability; once the penetration was accomplished by force, this requirement was legally satisfied.

The phrase "against her will" was interpreted by courts to mean without the consent of the woman.[6] If "illicit" intercourse was effected without force and with the consent of the woman, it might be adultery or fornication, but not rape. Consent was deemed to be absent when actual physical force was exercised on the body of the female or when threats of imminent physical harm were made to the woman by the rapist. Although this aspect of the law of rape varies widely from state to state, a lack of consent by the woman has also been found when the threats were made against the woman's child or relative or where the woman is deemed to be *legally* incapable of consenting to the act of intercourse because of a mental disease or defect, severe physical illness, or involuntarily induced unconsciousness because of alcohol or drugs.

To convict a defendant of rape, the government or prosecution had to prove all these elements: (1) illicit; (2) carnal knowledge; (3) of a female; (4) by force; and (5) against her will beyond a reasonable doubt. Unless that burden was met, the jury or fact finder was required by law to acquit or find the defendant "not guilty" of the charge of rape. Thus, in a courtroom and at law, the word *rape* is a legal conclusion. This is important because many victims, in answer to the question "What did the defendant do to you?" will respond, "He raped me." Since the *legal* question of whether or not a woman was raped is one for the jury to determine, the victim must describe exactly what the defendant did and not simply state the conclusion that she was raped. Although admittedly a technical point, it is one that upsets many victims. Further instructions and suggestions concerning tes-

---

[5]B. Manning, *The Criminal Offenses* (South Berlin, Mass.: Research Publishing Company, Inc., 1974), quoting *Commonwealth* v. *Goldenberg,* 338 Mass. 377, cert. den. 359, U.S. 1001 (1959), pp. 92, 104.
[6]Ibid. Quoting *Commonwealth* v. *Gardner,* 350 Mass. 664 (1966), pp. 93, 104; *Commonwealth* v. *Murphy,* 165 Mass. 66, 69 (1895).

tifying in court appear in Chapter 8; however, it is important here to emphasize to the victim that any courtroom objections to her use of the word *rape* in describing what happened to her does not mean either that people do not believe that she was raped or that the jury will not ultimately find her assailant guilty of the crime.

Legal Defenses to the Charge of Rape

Basically, there were at common law, and are now, two major legal defenses to the charge of rape. The first is called an *identification defense*. In this instance, the defendant, through his lawyer, usually concedes that the victim was "raped"—or, in other words, forced to have sexual intercourse with some male other than her husband against her will—but claims that he, the defendant, is not the male who raped her. This is essentially a defense of misidentification and is generally restricted to those instances where the victim and the rapist did not know each other prior to the rape and the victim subsequently identified the defendant through a lineup, police photographs, or some other identification procedure.

In the second typical kind of defense, the defendant will concede that he did have intercourse with the victim but will claim that the victim consented and that therefore the act of intercourse was not by force and against her will. This *consent defense* usually presents a much more difficult case for both the victim and the prosecution because ultimately it is the word of the victim against that of the defendant. Consent, if believed, constitutes a complete defense to the charge of rape. Of course, the jury may choose to disbelieve the defendant's contention that the victim consented, but, typically, it is the consent defense cases that cause the victim the most difficulty in the courtroom because both her conduct and, frequently, her entire lifestyle are under scrutiny.

Any male who is capable of penetrating the female vagina with his penis is legally capable of rape, and being a "juvenile" does not constitute a defense. A defendant who is below the maximum age for juvenile offenders (usually 16–18 years old) in the state where the rape occurred, however, will usually be tried in juvenile court. Most states have fairly strict rules regarding publicity in cases involving juvenile offenders, and the trial may be closed to the public. If convicted, the juvenile offender is usually confined in a juvenile detention facility rather than being sent to a state prison. In other regards, the legal process involving juveniles is essentially similar to that described for adult offenders.

Statutory Sexual Offenses

As state legislatures began to pass statutes forbidding certain types of conduct, common-law rape became part of state criminal laws and codes. In addition, most states enacted laws defining and punishing other types of sexually undesirable conduct as well.

One of the earliest and most common legislatively created sexual offenses was statutory rape, sometimes known as "abuse of a female child." In an effort to preserve and protect the chastity of young, impressionable females, many states made it a crime to have sexual intercourse with *any* female who was below the *legal* age of consent *regardless of whether she had consented to the intercourse.*[7] This age of consent varied, usually between 16 and 18 years of age. Following the common-law rule, if the underage female was legally married to the defendant, however, there could be no charge of statutory rape.

To prove a defendant guilty of this charge, the prosecution was required only to show that sexual intercourse occurred; it was not necessary to prove that the intercourse was against the will of the female. Furthermore, it was no defense to claim that the female had lied about her age, since at the time that most of these statutory rape laws were passed, it was a crime to engage in any sexual intercourse outside the bounds of legal marriage, and any person engaging in nonmarital sexual intercourse was on notice that such conduct was illegal.

Although in response to changing contemporary mores, most states have lowered the age of consent and/or the punishment for the offender if convicted, the crime of statutory rape exists today in almost all jurisdictions.

State legislatures also passed laws prohibiting and punishing sodomy, or anal intercourse, and oral sex, such as fellatio and cunnilingus. Often, in enacting these statutes, the legislatures used euphemistic language rather than describe the actual conduct prohibited. In Massachusetts, for example, sodomy was defined in the statute as an "abominable and detestable crime against nature";[8] the statute proscribing various types of oral sexual activity referred to "unnatural and lascivious acts."[9] Moreover, in many jurisdictions, the defendant could not raise a defense of consent even if the facts showed that the conduct occurred between "consenting" adults in private. In some instances, the defense of consent was legally unavailable even if the defendant was married to the "victim." The rationale underlying

[7]For an example, see Massachusetts General Law Annotated (MGLA), Chapter 265, Section 22 *et seq.*
[8]MGLA, Chapter 272, Section 34.
[9]MGLA, Chapter 272, Sections 35, 35A.

these statutes was that such conduct was repugnant to, as one court said, "the common sense of . . . decency, propriety and morality" of the community.[10]

Over time, legislatures and appellate courts defined these crimes more precisely, and many eventually permitted the defendant to raise the defense of consent if charged with the offense. However, in one form or another, these statutes are enforceable today. Unfortunately, many victims of sexual assault who are forced to commit sodomy, fellatio, or cunnilingus do not report these aspects of the incident to the police, either because they are too embarrassed or, possibly, because they do not realize that these acts constitute separate offenses apart from the "traditional" rape. Victims who do report to the police should be encouraged to include incidents of this type in their initial complaint, and medical personnel should be requested to gather evidence of these crimes in their examinations.

There are a wide variety of other sexual offenses as well. Among the most common of these are assault with intent to rape and indecent assault and battery. At common law, an *assault* was a threat to do bodily harm coupled with the present immediate ability to commit the harm threatened.[11] Thus, assault with intent to rape is a threat to commit rape, coupled with the present, immediate ability to commit the rape. *Battery*, at common law, was any unconsented-to, unjustified touching of the person of another.[12] *Indecent assault and battery* is, therefore, an immediate threat to do bodily harm, coupled with an actual touching or contact with the person of another in a manner that the legislature has defined as "indecent." What constitutes "indecent" in this context will differ from state to state but generally involves any unconsented-to, unjustified touching of the genital or breast area of a female. In some states, this crime is committed only if the victim of the assault and battery is under the age of consent or legally unable to consent.[13] Other modern statutory sexual offenses include: incestuous marriage or intercourse; inducing a "feebleminded" female to have intercourse; indecent assault and battery on a mentally retarded person; drugging a person for the purpose of having sexual intercourse; and "open and gross lewdness," which involves various types of sexual exhibitionism.

Modern Changes in the Law of Sexual Offenses

Until recently, most laws on sexual offenses presupposed by definition that the prohibited conduct was committed by a male against a female. In

[10]*Jaquith* v. *Commonwealth,* 331 Mass. 439, 443 (1954).
[11]Black, op cit., p. 147.
[12]Ibid., p. 193.
[13]For an example, see MGLA, Chapter 265, Sections 13B, 13F.

the past few years, a number of states have revised their criminal codes concerning sexual offenses. By using language such as "whoever commits a proscribed sexual offense against the person of another,"[14] these revised statutes now permit females as well as males to be charged with the offenses and provide the males as well as females may be the victims of such crimes. The legal definition of rape, in some states, has been expanded to include both sodomy and oral sex, as well as "digital" intercourse and the placing of foreign objects such as bottles and broomsticks in the vagina or the anus of the victim.[15]

The key to all these revisions seems to be the use of force by the assailant against the victim. Both courts and legislatures have recognized that certain conduct that was once forbidden, such as sodomy and oral sex between consenting adults, or intercourse with a 16-year-old girl, is now more widely accepted and practiced. However, when such conduct is accompanied by force and against the will of a person, regardless of the sex of the victim, legislatures have generally increased the penalties on conviction and frequently have provided for mandatory minimum sentences for repeated offenders.

Some states such as Wisconsin[16] have abolished many of the common-law and traditional statutory sexual offenses and replaced them with crimes describing different degrees of "sexual assault." Similar bills have been filed in the U.S. Congress and a number of state legislatures. Statutes of this type punish more severely those who commit the more violent types of sexual offenses, while attempting to provide lesser penalties for those who commit sexual offenses that are less obviously repulsive or violent.[17]

The aim is to give law enforcement personnel, judges, and juries greater flexibility in dealing appropriately with a variety of sexual offenses, and to encourage victims of different types of sexual assault to report these crimes.

Because of these changes, readers are urged to become familiar with the relevant law in their own state. The discussion of the criminal process that follows will assist those victims who decide to prosecute their cases in the criminal courts.

The Criminal Process

Paradoxically, while all victims of sexual assault are warned, encouraged, urged, and, occasionally, pressured into reporting the fact of their

[14]For an example, see MGLA, Chapter 265, Section 22ff.

[15]*Commonwealth* v. *Gallant,* 1977 Mass. Adv. Sh. 2254, 2263 (1977).

[16]Chapter 185, Laws of 1975 (State of Wisconsin, Senate Bill 233).

[17]See An Act to Amend Chapter 71 of Title 13 (Vermont, 1977); H.R. 4300 (U.S. Congress, 95th Session, 1977).

assault immediately, it is usually months before the case is actually tried. During this period, as discussed elsewhere in this book, many victims have been attempting to forget the incident and to proceed with their normal lives. Yet each time there is a required court appearance or, worse, an expected court appearance that does not happen, the victim is forced to remember and relive the incident again. The resulting anxiety and turmoil for the victim and the effects that this anxiety may have upon the victim's courtroom performance cannot be overstated. Not surprisingly, therefore, perhaps the question most frequently asked by victims is "Why does it take so long for my case to be tried?" Unfortunately, there is no simple or satisfactory answer to this question. To understand why this is so, a brief description of the criminal process as it functions in most states is necessary.

Although the time between arrest and trial varies from state to state and within states, in most urban areas, trials involving serious felonies like rape usually occur six months to a year after the crime was committed. There are many reasons for this delay, the primary being what is aptly called *court backlog.* The number of courtrooms, judges, and often prosecutors and defense lawyers is simply inadequate to provide trials for all persons accused of serious crimes. And since the rate of serious crime has been constantly rising, the problem gets worse every year.

However, even in those jurisdictions and states where case backlog is not the primary reason for delay, there are still a number of procedures, some of them required by the U.S. Constitution and individual state constitutions, that must be followed before a person may be tried for a serious crime.

First, a suspect, hereafter called a *defendant,* must be arrested. This may take time, especially if the victim and the defendant were strangers at the time of the rape. It may be necessary for the victim to look through police photographs, to attend lineups, or simply to wait until she sees the defendant again.

After the defendant is arrested, he is booked at a police station. Booking simply involves gathering certain data from the defendant, such as his address, birth date, and parents' names. He is then fingerprinted and photographed. Almost without exception, the victim is not present during these procedures. Identification by the victim occurs either before or after this process and is discussed in more detail in the next chapter. At the earliest opportunity, the arresting police officer or detective swears out a complaint against the defendant in the clerk's office for the judicial district where the rape occurred. The police officer swears out the complaint *on behalf of the state,* and he thus becomes the "complaining officer"; the victim is the "complaining witness." Since this procedure often causes confusion, it should be emphasized here that despite the victim's obvious involvement in the case, it is *not* the rape victim who brings charges; it is the state, government, commonwealth, etc., that is the moving party, and the case will always be referred to as, for example, the case of the *State* versus *John Smith.*

Arraignment

Following the issuance of a complaint, the defendant is arraigned in a district or other lower court. An arraignment is the formal process whereby a defendant is officially informed of the criminal charges against him. It consists of calling the defendant by name, in open court, reading the complaint to him, and asking him whether he wishes to plead guilty or not guilty. He is represented by counsel; if the defendant cannot afford to hire a lawyer, the judge will appoint one for him. Almost without exception, the defendant will plead not guilty. After the court clerk has entered the defendant's plea on the court papers, the judge will usually set bail or, in other words, decide how much money, if any, the defendant must produce before he will be released from custody. If the defendant does not have the necessary funds and cannot hire a bail bondsman to provide the money for him, he remains in custody. In most jurisdictions, the standards for the setting of bail, although not the specific dollar amount, are governed by statute.

It is *not* necessary for the victim to be present in court during the arraigment, although for a variety of reasons—some good and some not go good—she usually is. Since her presence in the courtroom can cause some legal problems later on in the process, *the victim should not go into the courtroom unless specifically instructed to do so by the arresting officer or the prosecutor in HER case.* If the victim is instructed to be at the courthouse and cannot find her arresting officer when she arrives, she should wait outside the courtroom until she sees him or should ask a supervising police officer (usually a police sergeant) for assistance in finding him.

Probable Cause Hearing

Many states have statutes or rules of court that require that a preliminary, or probable cause, hearing be held within a specified number of days after arraignment.

A probable cause hearing is a hearing and *not* a trial. There is no jury. A judge hears the facts, as testified to by witnesses under oath, and then decides whether those facts would cause a "reasonable, intelligent and prudent"[18] person to believe that it is more likely than not that the defendant has committed the crime for which he is charged—in this case, a rape.

---

[18]Black, op. cit., p. 1365.

The standard for this belief is not "beyond a reasonable doubt" but rather that there is enough evidence to make it likely or probable that he committed the crime. The defendant is under no obligation to present any kind of a defense and in most instances neither testifies nor calls any witnesses of his own.

The victim, on the other hand, must testify. And since her testimony is often taped or recorded by a stenographer, she should not testify unless she has talked to the prosecutor and is familiar with, at a bare minimum:

1. The time the rape occurred.
2. The place the rape occurred, including the lighting and identifiable objects such as furniture, trees, rocks, and buildings.
3. The means by which the rape occurred.
4. A description of the defendant as *he looked at the time of the incident,* including clothing, height, weight, build, age (estimates are all right), hair texture and color, eye color, and any other identifiable characteristics that she remembers.
5. Anything he said to her, including threats and statements about where he worked or lived.
6. How long the incident took.

Obviously, the victim must remember and be able to testify to the specific details of the incident; however, the most important rule for a successful rape prosecution is that there is absolutely no substitute for thorough and complete preparation. Some aids to assist the victim in "remembering" these details will be discussed in Chapter 8. At minimum, the victim can usually receive some assistance from the initial police report she gave of the incident (which is yet another reason that all rape victims should be encouraged to report the rape to the police immediately). The victim should also bring with her any tangible evidence that she may have saved.

Tangible evidence is anything that is capable of being felt or touched. In this instance, it would include ripped or bloody clothing or stockings; ropes, scarves, or anything that was used to bind her or gag her; and any other articles that were used either by her or the defendant during the incident, such as knives or paper. Some of these articles may have been given to the police—especially articles such as knives or paper that might contain fingerprints. Those articles will be kept by the police until the conclusion of the case.

It is very important that the victim save clothing and other tangible articles related to the rape. This fact cannot be stressed enough; as distasteful as it is, rape victims should not, under any circumstances, dispose of any article that might be tangible evidence.

The primary purpose of a probable cause hearing is to determine whether or not, at a threshold level, the police have arrested the right person. However, it also provides the defendant with an opportunity to find out the nature of the government's case against him; this process is called *discovery*. The defense lawyer can and will question the victim, often at length, and will use her answers in any subsequent jury trial. Lack of preparation will cause the victim difficulty at the probable cause hearing, and these problems will become compounded as the case moves through the system.

Despite the fact that court rules may require that the probable cause hearing be held within a specified number of days following arraignment, this rarely happens. Often, these hearings are rescheduled three or four times before the victim actually testifies. There are many reasons for these "continuances": sometimes the defendant does not have, or has not paid, his lawyer; sometimes either the defense lawyer or the prosecutor is occupied on other cases; sometimes the witnesses—including the victim—are unavailable; sometimes there are simply too many cases to be heard. Whatever the reason, the process is significantly delayed, often to the dismay of the victim.

Unfortunately, there is not much that the victim can do to speed the process. One suggestion that has been effective in many areas is to have the victim get the name and office phone of either her police officer or the prosecutor and to check *before* she comes to the courthouse to see if the case is actually going to be heard. Although the practice varies, usually the victim can be on "telephone call," which means that if she can be reached by telephone and can arrive at the courthouse within a half hour or so after being notified, she can go about her normal activities rather than having to sit at the courthouse waiting for her case to be reached. Before doing this, however, the victim/witness should always check with the police officer or the prosecutor. If she is unable to reach them, she should plan on being at the courthouse but should not sit in the courtroom unless instructed to do so by the police or the prosecutor.

Grand Jury

If, after hearing the evidence, the judge decides that there is probable cause to believe that the defendant has committed the rape, he will "bind the defendant over" for the grand jury. *Bind over* simply means that the defendant's case will be passed up to the next step in the process: the grand jury. The grand jury, an arm of the prosecutor's office, is composed of usually 16–23 people who hear evidence presented by the prosecutor and decide, by a majority vote, whether or not to indict the defendant. Many state constitutions require that a defendant be indicted before he can be tried for a felony. Since an indictment can be issued only by a grand jury, all rape cases proceed by way of a grand jury hearing in those jurisdictions that require indictment.[19]

There are two alternative methods to indictment by a grand jury. One is called *information* or, sometimes, a *bill of information*. An information, like an indictment, is an accusation based on probable cause; however, an information is filed on the oath of a "competent public official,"[20] usually a prosecutor, rather than on the oath of a majority of the grand jurors.

The other method is for the defendant to waive his right to have his case heard by a grand jury. This is known as *waiving indictment* and, in practice, occurs very infrequently. When it does happen, the choice is the defendant's and the victim is not a part of that process. The effect of waiving indictment is that the case usually proceeds to trial on the original complaint.

The standard used by the grand jury in deciding whether or not to indict a defendant is much the same as that used by the judge in the probable cause hearing: Is there probable cause to believe that the defendant committed the crime for which he is charged? However, the grand jury hears only one side of the case; except in rare instances, neither the defendant nor his lawyer is present. The victim may be asked to testify, but this time, she will be asked questions only by the prosecutor. It is a closed, or nonpublic, proceeding and the only persons present, aside from the members of the grand jury, are the prosecutor and a stenographer. Except when they are actually testifying, even the police officers are excluded. For most victims, the grand jury experience is a relatively easy one.

In many cases, however, the prosecutor who asks the questions in the grand jury is not the one who will try the victim's case before a jury. And since on any given day, the grand jury prosecutor may be presenting 10 or more different cases to the grand jury, the victim may not be able to confer with him or her before she testifies. The burden for remembering and preparing her testimony is on the victim.

Why, if the grand jury is not an adversary proceeding (i.e., the defense lawyer is not present), is it important for the witness to be just as well prepared as she was during the lower court hearing? The answer is that her testimony will be recorded by a stenographer, and at some time before the trial, the defense lawyer will ask for, and in many jurisdictions will receive, a transcript of her testimony before the grand jury. Once again, the better prepared she is for the grand jury, the easier it will be for her to prepare for the actual trial and the less likely it will be that she will become confused or forget important details. It should be noted here that some jurisdictions do

[19]Ibid., p. 912.
[20]Ibid., pp. 918–919.

not require that the rape victim actually testify before the grand jury.[21] In those instances, a police officer or counselor may be permitted to relate the facts of the incident to the Grand Jury.

If, after hearing the evidence presented, the Grand Jury decides that there is no probable cause to believe that the defendant has committed the rape for which he is charged, they will vote a "no bill," and the criminal process against the defendant ceases unless the prosecutor presents additional evidence that satisfies the grand jury. If, on the other hand, the grand jury believes that there is probable cause, it will vote a "true bill" (indictment), and the defendant will be held for trial by jury.

Some cases proceed to trial by way of a direct indictment. Since, in many jurisdictions, the defendant has no absolute right to a preliminary or probable cause hearing, the prosecutor may present the evidence directly to the grand jury—thus the term *direct indictment.* Because it prevents the discovery of the prosecution's case, which the preliminary hearing provides, many defense lawyers object to this method. Frequently, a prosecutor will proceed by way of a direct indictment when he/she wishes to avoid having the victim testify in the lower court. This procedure is especially useful when the victim is a young child who may forget the details of the incident if the case is not tried quickly or when the victim has been seriously injured or incapacitated by the rape. Increasingly, prosecutors are using direct indictments in cases of repeated or multiple offenders in an effort to bring the defendant to trial more rapidly. Whatever the reason, the obvious benefit to the victim is that the time between arrest and trial is greatly reduced. Although the decision to seek a direct indictment is ultimately the prosecutor's, counselors and/or parents of young victims should inquire about the possibility in those cases where a lengthy delay between arrest and trial would cause serious harm to the victim.

Following indictment, the defendant will be arraigned again, this time in the superior or other trial court. The victim is rarely present during arraignment in the trial court, and although the prosecutor usually notifies her, the victim's next *official* notification is by summons shortly before the case is scheduled to be tried. After arraignment, there may be a number of factors that delay the trial. The defense lawyer will probably file a number of pretrial motions, sometimes called *discovery motions.* Counsel may ask for all oral and written statements made by the defendant and the victim to the police and the prosecutor; he may also request to inspect the tangible evidence and conduct scientific tests. Once again, court rules determine how much time is permitted for these motions to be filed and answered, but

---

[21]Since "hearsay" testimony is permitted in a grand jury proceeding (see *Costello* v. *United States,* 350 U.S. 359, 76 S. Ct. 406 (1956), the decision as to whether or not any particular witness will be called to testify before the grand jury is, in the absence of a state statute, a matter of prosecutorial discretion.

delays, seemingly interminable to the victim, are not uncommon. While of little solace to the victim, the defendant is entitled to this information, and the trial cannot proceed until the defendant's discovery is complete.

Occasionally, the victim may be required to be present during some of these pretrial motions. A prosecutor or her police officer will usually contact her and ask her to come to the court if it is necessary for her to be there.

Finally, the case is scheduled to begin on a specific day. There are often delays because one of the lawyers is busy prosecuting or defending another case or the judge is in the midst of another trial on the day the victim's case was supposed to begin. Again, the best advice that can be given to the victim is to check with the prosecutor or the police officer before coming to court.

Trial

The trial of a felony case begins with the prosecutor's "moving for trial." This simply means that when everyone is ready, the prosecutor rises and informs the court that the State "moves" for trial on the indictment charging the defendant with rape. A group of potential jurors, sometimes called the *jury pool* or *venire*[22] is brought into the courtroom and asked questions to determine whether or not they will be impartial jurors. During the choosing, or empaneling, of a jury, the victim is generally not present in the courtroom. Once the jury is selected, the prosecutor makes an opening statement to the jury that briefly summarizes the government's case against the defendant. Following this opening, the prosecution calls its witnesses, including the victim, police officers, medical personnel, and other persons who either corroborate the victim's story or testify about aspects of the incident. After each witness is questioned by the prosecutor, the defense lawyer then questions, or cross-examines, the prosecution witnesses. When all prosecution witnesses have been questioned by both sides, the prosecution closes its case, or rests. Then the defendant may, if he chooses, present his witnesses and/or testify himself. The defense lawyer asks questions first, and when he/she is finished, the prosecution cross-examines the defense witnesses. *It should be emphasized here that the burden is on the prosecution to prove that the defendant is guilty beyond a reasonable doubt and that, as a matter of basic constitutional right, the defendant is not required to prove that he is innocent, to testify himself, or to call any witnesses on his own behalf.* The defense closes when all of the defendant's witnesses have been questioned by both sides.

After both sides rest, the evidence is closed and each lawyer makes a summation to the jury, or a closing argument. Each lawyer, by summariz-

22Black, op. cit., pp. 1726–1727.

ing the evidence most favorable to his/her side, tries to convince the jurors that they should either convict or acquit the defendant. When the lawyers have finished, the judge delivers the charge to the jury. The judge's remarks instruct the jury about the principles of law that they must apply in reaching a verdict. The jury then leaves the courtroom to decide, or deliberate on, its verdict.

Whether or not the victim is present in the courtroom during the trial depends either on personal preference or on a court ruling. Some victims want to hear the entire case; others want to leave as soon as they are finished testifying. In some instances, however, the judge issues an *order of sequestration,* which means that all witnesses in a case are excluded from the courtroom during the trial except when they are actually testifying. If a judge issues such an order, the victim may not remain in the courtroom during the trial, although she probably will be permitted to hear the closing arguments and the judge's instructions to the jury.

A jury verdict in a criminal felony case must be unanimous. If a jury is unable to agree unanimously about whether the defendant is guilty or not guilty, it is known as a *hung jury* and the case must be tried again. When a jury does reach a unanimous decision, they return to the courtroom and report their verdict. If the defendant is found not guilty, he is discharged by the judge and is free to leave. If he is convicted, he will generally be sentenced to state prison.

Following a guilty verdict, the defendant has a right to appeal his conviction to an appellate court. There are no juries in an appellate court, and the victim is not required to testify or even be present. The case is argued to a panel of judges after both sides have submitted written reports, or briefs, to the judges. The appellate court will either uphold the conviction or reverse the conviction. If the conviction is reversed, the defendant is usually entitled to another trial.

The criminal process described varies from state to state. It is often exceedingly slow and, to many rape victims, infuriatingly so; however, an understanding of the process and some of the reasons for the delays, coupled with a sensitive and commonsense approach about when the victim should actually appear in court, may enable her to deal more effectively with the often-expressed sentiment that her case has been "forgotten" or that "nobody cares" what happens to her and her case.

The Issue of Bail

Until recently, most persons accused of serious felonies remained in custody until their trial. Since the mid-1960s, however, many states have enacted bail reform statutes to prevent lengthy pretrial detention. These statutes favor admitting a defendant to bail *provided* he can demonstrate to the court's satisfaction that he has the necessary "strong community ties" (e.g., has lived in the community for an extended period, holds a job, and has family in the vicinity to ensure that, if released, he will be unlikely to flee the jurisdiction).[23] The judge considers the nature of the crime, the defendant's previous criminal record, and the strength of his community ties in determining the setting of bail, which may range from personal recognizance to very high dollar amounts. If the defendant can either raise the required money himself or hire a bail bondsman to issue a bond guaranteeing his reappearance, he will be released.[24] If not, he remains in custody in lieu of bail until the case is tried.

For many rape victims, the fact that the assailant is released on bail rather than being held in custody awaiting trial is very disturbing. Some victims believe that the attacker will return, especially if he had initially threatened reprisals if she went to the police. Others imagine that they are being followed or fear that their normal lives will be disrupted even further by phone calls or threats from the defendant released on bail. While the actual likelihood of a defendant's harrassing a victim is slight, it is important to remember that the admitting of a defendant to bail is never final; a defendant's bail can be increased or even revoked entirely if new information about the defendant and his conduct is brought to the attention of the judge who originally set the bail. Obviously, intimidating, threatening, or harrassing a victim is "new" information and should be brought to the court's attention as soon as possible. Most judges regard the harrassment of witnesses as an extremely serious matter, and all victims should be encouraged to report such conduct to the police or the prosecutor.

The following suggestions may help to reduce some of the victim's anxiety about future or potential dangers if the defendant is released on bail:

1. The arresting police officer or prosecutor should be told *immediately* about any actual harrassment, threats, or comments directed toward the victim, her family, or her friends by either the defendant himself or any of his friends or relatives. The victim should be as specific as possible concerning who made the threats, what was said or done, where the threat or harrassment occurred, and who else was present. If the victim is unable to contact the police immediately, she should write down the specific details as soon as practicable so that she will not forget them.

2. If the victim reasonably suspects that someone is following her or if she is receiving anonymous phone calls, she should keep a log of the date, time, and place and then call her police officer or prosecutor. Changing or

[23] For an example, see MGLA, Chapter 276, Section 58.
[24] Black, op. cit., p. 177.

unlisting a phone number is another possibility, although generally the local phone company will charge for this service. The police may be of some assistance in expediting the process and, in some instances, can even arrange for a waiver of the normal charge.

3. If the rape did not occur in the victim's home and/or she has moved since the incident and she does not wish to have her current address known, she should tell the police and the prosecutor, and, in most instances, her specific address can be omitted from court proceedings and documents.

4. Since the victim will probably be apprehensive when she learns that the defendant has been released on bail, she should be encouraged not to travel alone, especially at times and in locations where she might encounter the defendant. Although this is usually an unnecessary precaution, it may spare the victim an unpleasant confrontation.

Whatever the real or imagined concerns of the victim, it is crucial to emphasize that her conduct should be guided by a healthy dose of common sense. The defendant is not entitled to bail; it is a privilege that can be revoked if abused. The victim should be encouraged in believing that the defendant will not attempt to intimidate or harrass her, but if he or someone connected with him does bother her, she should not hesitate to contact the police or the prosecutor.

Summary

Rape and related sexual offenses are serious felonies. Although the specific elements necessary to be proved may vary, the criminal justice system deals severely with those who have been convicted. Modern criminal statutes prohibit and punish many different types of aberrant and/or violent sexual conduct, and victims of sexual attacks should be encouraged to report these offenses to the police.

Because rape and related sexual offenses are such serious felonies, all the various constitutional and procedural guarantees of due process and a fair trial apply to the prosecution and conviction of persons accused of these offenses. While some of these guarantees result in a very lengthy criminal process that may cause anxiety and frustration for the victim, these delays are frequently the unavoidable result of basic constitutional rights that form the foundation of our system of government. Ultimately, it is better for the individual victim, as well as for our entire system of criminal justice, that the defendant be prosecuted and convicted according to law. Patience and an understanding of the process may help the sexual assault victim to cope with what often seem to be interminable delays in her case and may help her not to personalize criminal justice procedures.

8

The Experience of the Rape Victim
in the Courtroom

ALICE E. RICHMOND

Every weekday, in criminal courts throughout the United States, literally thousands of people are involved in the trial of criminal cases. Yet, most victims of sexual assault have had no previous contact with the criminal justice system. Suddenly they find themselves participants in a process in which they understand neither the rules nor the roles of the other participants. The entire environment is intimidating, and the fact that in most jurisdictions the vast majority of participants are male may add to the victim's apprehension and discomfort.

Compounding the confusion is the victim's often-expressed complaint that "No one tells me what I am supposed to do." Although the sensitivity of participants in the system to the peculiar problems of rape victims is improving, this complaint is understandable. The victim is asked to testify and to describe events and circumstances that are embarrassing and painful and to do so in a large, public courtroom where she is often subjected to difficult cross-examination by the defendant's lawyer. The victim may have questions about whether she will be required to testify about her past sexual conduct, about how she should dress and act on the witness stand, and about what she should do if she forgets something. She may wonder about the roles of the other participants in the trial, her relationship to them, and, especially, if her attacker will be present when she testifies.

This chapter will attempt to answer these questions, although a note of caution is necessary. The experience of individual victims varies depending on a number of factors. A victim who has a good relationship with the

ALICE E. RICHMOND, Esq. ● Former Assistant District Attorney, Suffolk District; former Assistant Professor, New England School of Law, Boston, Massachusetts.

investigating police officer and the prosecutor will usually have an easier, less unpleasant experience as a witness. And while many states now mandate the training of police and prosecutors in rape sensitivity courses, many jurisdictions do not.[1] Moreover, the fact that an officer or a prosecutor has been "sensitized" in a classroom setting does not guarantee that he or she will deal effectively with any given rape victim.

The courtroom experience of victims is to some degree a function of the specific facts of the case. For example, a woman who is raped in her home at 8 A.M. by a perfect stranger will generally have an easier time in the courtroom than a woman who, to use the vernacular, picked up a man in a singles' bar and invited him back to her apartment at 2 A.M. in the morning. This is not to imply that the "singles' bar" rape is not as vicious or violent as the "stranger" rape. But, in the former example, the defense, as noted in Chapter 7, will probably revolve around the "identification" of the defendant, and questioning about the assault itself will be minimal.

Finally, police officers, prosecutors, juries, and judges reflect the attitudes and prejudices of the larger society. A woman who was hitchhiking or in a bar alone at the time she was assaulted will probably feel less sympathy from the participants than a woman whose conduct is viewed as less contributory to the assault. Juries traditionally do not like to convict a defendant of a serious crime solely on the uncorroborated word of another human being. For a rape victim, in a case where the defendant raises a defense of consent, this fact is especially relevant.

Victims and counselors should attempt to familiarize themselves with specific procedures in their own jurisdictions. This chapter identifies in general terms the participants in the courtroom process and provides the victim/witness with suggestions about appropriate conduct and responses during a jury trial.

The Role of the Prosecutor and Witness Preparation

Many rape victims wonder if they must hire a lawyer to represent their interests in court. The answer to this question, except in the most unusual circumstances, is no. Although the actual rape was committed against an individual, the crime itself is considered, at law, a crime against the "peace, order and stability" of the entire society.[2] For this reason, rape cases are

---

[1] National Institute of Law Enforcement and Criminal Justice, *Forcible Rape: Police Volume 1* (1977), p. 34. For an example, see Chapter 581 of the Acts and Resolves of 1974 Amending Massachusetts General Laws Annotated (MGLA), Chapters 6 (Sections 118, 156), 41 (Section 97B), and 280 (Section 2).

[2] H. C. Black, *Black's Law Dictionary* (revised 4th ed.) (St. Paul, Minn.: West Publishing Company, 1968), pp. 444–445.

presented in court by a public prosecutor, who is also known as a district attorney, a state's attorney, or an attorney general.

In geographically large or heavily populated areas, the prosecuting attorney will probably be called an assistant district attorney or assistant state's attorney. The designation *assistant* does not mean that the victim's case is being relegated to a less competent or qualified lawyer. In most areas, the district or state attorney is an elected official. Since the volume of cases to be tried is too great for one person, the elected official is permitted to hire "assistants" to help prosecute the cases in court.

Jurisdictions do differ in the method by which cases are assigned to individual prosecutors for trial. Generally, however, rape cases are assigned to the more experienced prosecutors. Once a case has been assigned to a specific prosecutor for trial, it is the attorney's responsibility to organize the case and prepare the witnesses for trial.

Some prosecutor's offices function on a vertical model. This means that the same prosecutor will handle the case from the time a complaint is sworn out against the defendant in the lower court through the trial and, perhaps, even to the appellate level if the defendant is convicted. Other offices assign some prosecutors to handle only preliminary hearings and have a different set of prosecutors assigned to the grand jury and the trial court. Thus, some victims may have as many as three prosecutors during the course of their case. In some instances, such as when the victim is a child or the particular facts of the case warrant it, either the victim or her counselor should request that the same prosecutor be assigned the case throughout its course. Where possible, most prosecutors' offices will attempt to accommodate the victim.

In the event that the victim must cooperate with different prosecutors, it is useful to bring a complete, *written* statement of the facts to the initial interview. Although the "new" prosecutor will want to ask some questions, the victim will probably not have to repeat the details of the entire incident.

Although in *every* rape case the victim must identify the defendant as the person who raped her, pretrial identification procedures will be used only in those cases where the victim and the defendant were strangers at the time of the rape. In these cases, if the defendant was not caught during or immediately after the crime occurred, it is necessary for the victim to identify the defendant, either through pictures and/or in person after he is arrested. Sometimes the police officers will come to the victim's home and show her a book or group of photographs. Frequently, the victim is asked to come to the police station or the courthouse to view these photographs. Despite the fact that no testimony is given, these visits are crucial to the prosecution of her case.

Once the suspect has been arrested, the victim will be asked to identify him in person. In some instances, this in-person identification is done through the use of a lineup. A number of men (usually no less than five), who all fit the description given by the victim at the time of the incident, will be literally lined up in a room. The victim can look at all of them, in profile or full view, and can request that they all be asked to say a certain phrase or word. After she has had an opportunity to view all of them, she will be asked by the prosecutor or the police whether or not she can identify any of them. If the lineup occurs in a police station, it is likely that the victim will view the men through a special mirrorlike glass. She will be able to see into the room where the men are standing, but they will see only a mirror image of themselves on the other side. If the lineup occurs in a courtroom or if the victim is present in the same room as the defendant, then he will be able to see her.

More frequently, however, there is neither the time nor the resources for a lineup, and the in-person identification occurs in the courtroom before the arraignment or the preliminary hearing. The rules governing how a victim may identify her assailant in a courtroom situation are determined by the constitutional guarantees of due process and the right to counsel. Inherent in these guarantees is the idea that seeing a defendant in custody, or in handcuffs, may lead a witness to make an incorrect or mistaken identification. Or, to phrase it another way, seeing a person alone in a prisoner's dock, after being told by the police that the defendant is in the courtroom, is so inherently suggestive that any identification by the victim that takes place under these circumstances is unconstitutional and therefore inadmissible at the trial. For this reason, police officers will often not tell a rape victim why they want her to come to court. The victim should always find her police officer or prosecutor before she goes into the courtroom for the first time and follow his instructions carefully. It is not that the police or the prosecutor doubts the victim's ability to identify the defendant; rather, it is that by following the required procedures, the prosecution can avoid any later charge that the initial in-person identification was unconstitutionally suggestive or otherwise improper.

The victim may also be asked to come to court for witness preparation. This is an opportunity for the victim to speak with the prosecutor, to ask any questions she may have about the procedure or trial, and to become familiar with what will be expected from her in the courtroom. Many victims express their feelings about the actual incident by saying, "I just didn't feel as if I had any control over what was happening to me." With adequate witness preparation, this feeling of helplessness will not be repeated during the trial.

In a very real sense, witness preparation begins immediately after the incident. The very first thing a rape victim should do is to tell the police, a close friend, a relative, or a counselor *everything* that she can remember about the incident. Although this may be psychologically uncomfortable for the victim, it is important that this be done immediately for two reasons.

Over time, specifics of the incident will fade and important details may be forgotten. In many rape cases, especially those in which the defendant's arrest occurred some days or even weeks after the incident, the initial description of both the defendant and the circumstances of the assault is an issue at the trial. Furthermore, these initial reports will not only aid the victim in refreshing her memory before the trial but provide corroboration for her in-court testimony. This corroboration is known as *fresh complaint* and is the single most useful aid in the prosecution of the victim's case.

What is *fresh complaint?* Simply stated, it is an exception to the Hearsay Rule that permits a police officer, friend, relative, or counselor to testify in court as to the specific details that the victim reported about the rape, provided that the victim made these statements as soon after the incident as possible, usually not more than 24 hours after the incident occurred.

The sole purpose of the fresh complaint exception is to permit witnesses *other than the victim* to corroborate her in-court testimony by repeating what she said to them immediately after the incident. In cases where it is simply the victim's word against the defendant's, a fresh complaint witness can be the difference between conviction and acquittal. The victim who does not report her rape to the police or tell anyone about it for several days is obviously at a disadvantage should she later decide to prosecute, since this doctrine of fresh complaint is unavailable to corroborate her testimony.

Even if the victim does report the rape immediately, she should also write her own notes of the incident as soon as possible. Again, these will be an aid to her in preparing for trial and in discussing her case with the prosecutor. Unfortunately, the reports received by the prosecutor before he/she actually interviews the victim are often incomplete. The victim's own report can thus be of assistance to the prosecutor in identifying and locating evidence and witnesses.

Although witness preparation varies, most prosecutors use the preparation session to give the victim some hints about testifying and to explain what she can expect from the defense lawyer when he/she is cross-examining her. The prosecutor may also ask some rather pointed questions about what appear to be problems with the case. The victim should not assume that these questions mean that the prosecutor does not believe her story. A prosecutor must make reasoned decisions about trial tactics and legal strategy based on a professional evaluation of the strength of any given case. It is always preferable for the prosecutor to know and prepare for these problems before the case is called for trial rather than to be surprised by some fact while the trial is actually in progress.

Finally, the victim should realize that she might not be in the best position to make a realistic evaluation of her case and the amount of time needed for trial preparation. The police and the prosecutors assume that given a choice, the victim would prefer not to be subjected to the criminal justice process, and they usually try to minimize the inconvenience and unpleasantness for her. However, a successful prosecution is almost always a result of good preparation, and witness cooperation can only aid the prosecutor in presenting her case to the jury.

The Role of the Defense Lawyer and Cross-Examination

The right of a criminal defendant to confront and question all witnesses testifying for the prosecution is guaranteed by the Sixth Amendment to the U.S. Constitution.[3] Therefore, the questioning of the sexual assault victim by the defendant's lawyer is an essential and immutable part of her court-room experience. For many victims, this questioning, or cross-examination, is the most dreaded aspect of the entire judicial process. An impression shared by many, if not all, victims who have testified in court is that the defense lawyer was out to get her or was trying to trick her or make a fool of her.

Hours could be spent arguing about why someone would defend a rapist and, even if one did, why it is necessary to question the victim in the aggressive manner employed by many defense lawyers. Suffice it to say here that every person accused of a crime, no matter how heinous, is enti-tled to be represented by competent counsel, who is expected to perform to the best of his or her abilities. Furthermore, the central issue at any trial is the *credibility* of the witnesses. Thus, the primary job of the defense lawyer is to show that the victim is either not telling the truth about the incident or that she is mistaken about the details (such as the description of the defend-ant, the time, and the place) that connect the commission of the rape with his/her client. The tactics used by defense lawyers vary, but to the victim, these tactics often seem hostile.

The particular manner in which a victim is questioned depends on the skill and personality of the individual defense lawyer. Admittedly, some defense lawyers try to upset or rattle the witness through tone of voice and innuendo; others hammer away at seemingly insignificant details. What-ever his/her style, the victim should try to remember that the defense lawyer is only doing his/her job, and his/her challenges to her testimony should not be taken personally.

[3]The Constitution of the United States, Amendment VI, states in its entirety: "In all criminal prosecutions, the accused shall enjoy the right to a speedy and public trial, by an impartial jury of the state and district wherein the crime shall have been committed, which district shall have been previously ascertained by law, and to be informed of the nature and cause of the accusation; to be confronted with the witnesses against him; to have compulsory process for obtaining Witnesses in his favor, and to have the Assistance of Counsel for his defence."

The tendency of many victims to view the cross-examination as a frontal attack on their truthfulness is widespread and understandable. However, if the victim is well-prepared, she will remember the necessary details. There will be other evidence—for example, hospital reports, torn clothing, and fresh complaint witnesses—that corroborate her testimony. Furthermore, the defense lawyer must abide by the rules of evidence, and in most jurisdictions, the judge, on proper objection from the prosecutor, excludes questions that are "argumentative," and the victim is not required to respond to the question.

One of the fundamental principles of cross-examination is the use of leading questions, and thus victims should understand how to recognize and how to answer this type of inquiry. Essentially, a leading question is a question that, by its phrasing, suggests an answer and usually must be answered by either a "yes" or a "no"; failure to respond with either a "yes" or a "no" may result in the witness's answers being excluded as "nonresponsive."

For example, suppose that on direct examination by the prosecutor, the victim testified that the rape occurred at about 5:00 P.M. on January 7 at the corner of Spring and Winter Streets. On cross-examination, the defense lawyer may ask, "You've testified that this incident occurred on January 7th at the corner of Spring and Winter Streets at about 6:00 P.M., is that correct?" The natural inclination of most witnesses is to say, "Yes," since most of the facts contained in the question are correct; however, the defense lawyer has suggested that the rape took place at 6:00 P.M. and not 5:00 P.M. This apparent misstatement may have been unintentional; however, it is more likely that the defense lawyer has a particular reason for wanting to establish that the rape occurred at 6:00 P.M. instead of 5:00 P.M. In any event, the victim, by answering "yes" to the question, has now introduced an inconsistency in her testimony that may become more important later in the case, especially if other witnesses testify that she reported that the rape occurred at 5:00 P.M. and the defendant has an alibi starting at 6:00 P.M. In this example, the only appropriate answer to the defense lawyer's question would be "no."

Since this type of question is perfectly proper, the witness must be prepared for such questions and know how to answer them. The basic rule is for the witness to listen very carefully to the entire question and to take her time in answering. She should never assume that the question being asked is unimportant and simply a restatement of previous testimony. If the victim does not understand the question, she can and should ask the defense lawyer to repeat it. If any part of the question is incorrect, such as in the example given above, she should answer "no" and wait for the next question.

The defense lawyer may ask the rape victim a question to which she does not know the answer. Or he/she may ask her a question about something that she cannot recall. A witness is expected to testify to the best of her memory; if she has forgotten or does not know an answer, it is perfectly proper for her to respond, "I don't know" or "I can't recall." Again, good witness preparation will prevent some of these problems. It is important to remember that it is never a good idea to guess at an answer. Often, in guessing at an answer, the victim will contradict the testimony of another prosecution witness. Thus, regardless of how many times a particular question is asked, if the witness honestly does not know the answer, or cannot now recall the answer, she should not be pressured into guessing regardless of the tone of voice or persistence of the cross-examiner.

Another area that frequently causes problems for witnesses involves testimony about time, distances, and descriptive details such as height and weight. In normal conversation, people almost always speak in terms of approximations. For example, "I got to the office about 4:30 or 4:45" or "He was approximately 5'6" tall" or "He weighed about 200 pounds" or "It was about 50 or 60 feet away." Yet, many witnesses feel that they must be more specific in the courtroom, especially if the defendant's lawyer begins to question them closely about these normal approximations. Often, in response to intense questioning, witnesses will concede 1 or 2 inches on height or 10 or 15 feet on distance or an hour on time.

Sometimes these details are insignificant in the jury's determination of the defendant's guilt or innocence. Occasionally, however, these concessions are dispositive of the case, especially if the defendant convinces the jury that he was somewhere else when the crime was committed or is of a different height than that finally testified to by the victim, or that there are so many inconsistencies in the witness's testimony that she should not be believed. The answer to this common dilemma is quite simple: in answering questions about time, distance, or descriptive details, witnesses should *always* use approximations and use them consistently throughout the trial. The exception would be if the victim is positive about the details, for example, "It was 9:30 P.M. when I first saw the defendant. I know that because I had just looked at my watch."

Another typical area of inquiry involves whether or not the victim has talked to the police or the prosecutor and has gone over her testimony with them. Many witnesses feel that this is a question that they must answer in the negative. The prevailing logic seems to be that if the jury hears that the witness has discussed her testimony ahead of time, they will feel that somehow she has been unfairly prepared for trial. This perception is incorrect; whenever the witness is asked a question of this type, she should answer that she *has* discussed her testimony with the police or the prosecutor and has done so, if this is the case, on a number of occasions. Almost invariably, the next question from the defendant's lawyer will be "And they told you what to say, didn't they?" or sometimes, "What did they tell you to say?" The answer from the victim to this line of inquiry should be "No" or "They told me to tell the truth." There is nothing improper in discussing testimony with the prosecutor or the police officers assigned to the case; in fact, it is expected. The witness should always be prepared to answer these questions directly; to do otherwise jeopardizes her credibility.

For many victims of a sexual assault, the most dreaded area of inquiry on cross-examination concerns their prior sexual conduct or evidence about their "sexual reputation." This is especially true when the victim is young or unmarried. Theoretically, evidence of a victim's prior sexual reputation or conduct can be presented either by questioning her on cross-examination or by offering testimony through a witness called by the defense. In the vast majority of cases involving sexual assault, evidence of this type is either legally immaterial or legally insufficient and therefore inadmissible. Because so many sexual assault victims refuse to prosecute their assailants in court because they are afraid or embarrassed about being questioned on this subject, it might be useful to understand the requirements for the admission of this type of evidence.

Admissibility of Sexual History Testimony

As noted previously, the presentation of testimony during a hearing or a trial is governed by the rules of evidence. These rules require that *all* testimony elicited from all the witnesses be legally "material" or "relevant" to the actual case being tried. Information is considered material if it tends to have a "legitimate and effective influence or bearing" on the way the case is decided by a judge or jury.[4] Testimony, even if true, that is collateral to the main issue in the trial (in this instance, whether the defendant raped the victim) and that will tend to confuse or divert the fact finder from a fair determination of this central issue is excluded from evidence as immaterial or irrelevant.

Thus, when the victim herself is asked about her previous sexual experience or conduct by a defense lawyer, the prosecutor can object to the question, and the burden is then on the defense lawyer to show that the victim's answer is relevant to the determination of the defendant's guilt or innocence. The mere fact that a victim has had an abortion, is taking birth control pills or was not a virgin at the time of the rape is not generally relevant, and any questions asked of her in an attempt to elicit this information before a jury will be ruled immaterial and therefore inadmissible. In other words, the victim may not be required to answer the question. Victims

4Black, op. cit., p. 1128.

should remember, however, that while a judge may rule that a victim does not have to answer a particular question, nothing prevents or prohibits the defense lawyer from *asking* the question.

There are situations in which the victim's prior sexual conduct and experience may be relevant at trial. For instance, any prior sexual involvement with the defendant usually *is* admissible, and the victim should expect to have to testify about it. Also, her sexual conduct in the day or two preceding the rape may be ruled material if there has been medical testimony that sperm were found in the victim's vagina after the assault, since the presence of sperm could be the result of earlier voluntary intercourse rather than the result of rape.

One further qualification is necessary. In many jurisdictions, questions to the victim concerning her prior sexual conduct are not admissible (even if the answer might be material) in the absence of a good faith belief by defense counsel that the victim did indeed engage in voluntary intercourse during some period relevant to the trial. To put it more bluntly, defense counsel is not permitted to conduct the proverbial fishing expedition by asking questions concerning the victim's prior sexual experience with a hope that some material fact may be discovered.

Many sexual assault victims are afraid that information about their sexual history and experience will be presented through defendant's witnesses who will testify about the victim's sexual reputation. While there is such a concept as *reputation evidence,* the requirements governing its admissibility are widely misunderstood, and it is infrequently used in rape cases.[5] An explanation of the nature and requirements of reputation evidence might serve to minimize victim concern about this type of testimony.

In most jurisdictions, testimony about specific instances of prior sexual conduct or history is generally inadmissible. More importantly, the use of reputation evidence usually requires more than simply calling some witness who claims to have information about the victim's prior sexual conduct. Before such a witness may testify, the defense lawyer must show that the victim had, at the time of the attack, a reputation in the community for sexual promiscuity.[6] To do this, the defense lawyer must locate a person who knows the victim and will testify under oath that (1) he has lived or worked in the same community as the victim for an extended period of time; (2) that he has heard from other people in this same community that the victim has a reputation in this community concerning her sexual conduct based on a number of incidents or recurring patterns; (3) that he has heard the victim's reputation discussed on a number of occasions; and (4) that the victim's reputation in the community as discussed by members of this community and heard personally by this witness is one of sexual promiscu-

[5]Ibid., pp. 1467–1468.
[6]Ibid., pp. 1467–1468.

ity. Furthermore, even if the defense can find such a person willing and able to so testify, the ultimate test governing the admissibility of this evidence is again materiality or relevancy.

Cases where evidence of a rape victim's reputation for sexual promiscuity has been introduced have primarily involved situations where the victim and the defendant knew each other prior to the alleged rape and where the defendant is offering a defense of consent. Because of the difficulty in establishing the necessary legal foundation for the admissibility of reputation evidence, it is generally limited to consent defense cases occurring in rural or nonurban areas; in an urban setting, it is extremely difficult to establish that a victim has a well-known and long-standing reputation in the community for sexual promiscuity.

Despite these limitations and the difficulty of introducing evidence concerning the victim's prior sexual history, recent studies have confirmed that significant numbers of victims either fail to report their attacks to the police or refuse to prosecute after the assailant has been arrested because of fear and embarrassment about being questioned about their previous sexual history.[7] To encourage more victims of sexual assault to report the incidents and prosecute their assailants in court, a number of state legislatures as well as the U.S. Congress (P.L. 95-540) have enacted statutes that regulate the admissibility of evidence of the victim's sexual conduct in sexual assault cases. Although the specific provisions of these statutes vary from state to state, they usually include strong language *excluding* evidence of specific instances of the victim's sexual conduct except in very limited circumstances. Some examples of instances when such evidence might be admissible include: "(1) evidence of the victim's sexual conduct with the defendant; (2) evidence of the recent conduct of the victim tending to explain the source of any physical feature, characteristic, or condition of the victim; and (3) when the judge finds that such evidence is relevant to a fact at issue and that its prejudicial nature does not outweight its probative value."[8]

Some statutes also include specific procedures for the defense lawyer wishing to offer evidence of the victim's prior sexual conduct. A request in the form of a written motion containing the facts that the defense lawyer expects to elicit from the victim must be made to the judge before the offering of any evidence of this type. In statutes containing this requirement, the hearing is held *in camera,* out of the hearing of the jury, and may occur in the judge's private chambers, to minimize embarrassment to the victim.[9] It is only after this proceeding, and if the judge finds that the exceptions to the statute apply, that the victim may be asked questions

[7]*Forcible Rape,* op. cit.
[8]MGLA, Chapter 233, Section 21B; H.R. 408 (U.S. Congress, 95th Session, 1977).
[9]MGLA, Chapter 233, Section 21B.

about her prior sexual history in open court and then only in the limited areas already approved by the judge.

The effectiveness of these statutes is still difficult to determine since most have been enacted recently. It is hoped that such provisions will be useful in encouraging wider reporting and prosecuting of sexual assault cases.

By making it a matter of public policy that evidence of a victim's prior sexual history is inappropriate in a sexual assault trial except in very limited circumstances, notice has been served not only to victims of sexual assault but to all other participants in the system that it is no longer open season on sexual assault victims in the courtroom. As of 1979, relatively few states had enacted statutes of this type. Persons involved in the counseling of sexual assault victims should attempt to learn whether such statutes have been enacted in their jurisdictions. If they have not, action should be taken to investigate the possibility of proposing such legislation through their local state representatives and senators.

The Role of the Judge

In simplest terms, the role of the trial judge is to be an impartial person who, through his or her rulings on the admissibility of evidence and interpretation of the applicable law, controls the progress of a trial. Since our judicial system is, by definition, an adversary system, the judge acts as referee between the parties. Because the judge's allegiance is to neither side, the judge ensures that both sides will have an equal opportunity to present their case in court consistent with the rules of evidence and relevant statutes and laws.

One way in which the judge referees is through rulings on objections to testimony and real evidence. Suppose that during the prosecutor's questioning of the victim, the defense counsel stands and objects either to the prosecutor's question or to the victim's answer. The judge must decide whether the objected-to question and/or answer is correct as to form or content. If the judge sustains the objection, then the question asked or the answer given will be excluded; occasionally, if an improper question has already been answered by the witness, the answer will be stricken and the jury instructed to disregard the answer.

Unfortunately, many witnesses assume that the sustaining of an objection by the judge means that the witness has done or said something improper. This is rarely the case, especially if the objection was made to an improper question. For this reason, among others, witnesses should always try to wait until a judge has ruled on an objection before answering a question. If the judge says that the objection is overruled, then the witness may answer the question. If the witness is uncertain about the judge's ruling, it is perfectly proper for the witness to ask the judge whether or not the question should be answered.

The more difficult problem emerges when the witness's answer is objected to and stricken. Generally, there are two major reasons for striking an answer: (1) it is unresponsive to the question (Question: "What did you do then?" Answer: "I thought he was going to kill me"); or (2) sometimes the witness has answered the question responsively but has done so in an inadmissible form (Question: "What happened then?" Answer: "He raped me." Since, as mentioned previously, rape is a legal conclusion, the victim must describe what the defendant actually did). In either event, the witness is often confused about what she did wrong and assumes that the *content,* as opposed to the form, of her answer is incorrect.

The alert witness may be able to determine what the problem is simply by listening to the words used by the lawyer when the objection is made. For example, the lawyer may say, "Your honor, I move to strike; the answer is nonresponsive." The witness should then try to rephrase her answer in a more specific manner. A witness may generally assume that if a question is repeated by the questioning counsel essentially *verbatim,* then it is the way in which she answered the question, rather than the content of her answer, that is objectionable. If, however, the witness is unable to determine why her answer to a given question has been stricken, then it is perfectly proper to indicate to the questioning lawyer, or to the judge, that she is uncertain about how to answer the question. Very often, a judge may rephrase the question by asking the witness a different question, which in his/her discretion, need not follow the rules of evidence.

Although the victim should not be afraid to ask the judge a question when she does not understand what is happening, a cautionary note is necessary. Judges, because they are impartial, cannot and should not be expected to provide solace and support to the victim during her testimony. Too many victims assume that the judge's facial expression or conduct during testimony is an indication of approval or disapproval. Furthermore, since most trial judges take notes during a trial, some victims assume that if the judge appears to be constantly taking notes, the trial is proceeding better than if he/she is not. The victim should simply be reminded that her attention should be on the lawyers and the jury unless she has a specific problem that relates to her conduct as a witness.

Following the testimony of all the witnesses and closing arguments by both the prosecutor and the defense counsel, the judge will deliver the charge to the jury. A charge is an explanation of the law and the requirements that a jury must follow in reaching a verdict. During the charge, only the judge speaks, and in many jurisdictions, once the judge has started speaking, no one is permitted to leave or enter the courtroom.

Occasionally, a sexual assault case may be tried jury-waived which means that the *defendant* has waived his right to be tried by a jury and chooses instead to have the trial judge be the fact finder in deciding on his guilt or innocence. Since the right to a trial by jury in a felony case is one of our basic constitutional guarantees, it may *only* be waived knowingly and intelligently by the defendant; the victim and the prosecutor have no role in this decision. Since jury-waived sexual assault cases are relatively rare, victims should request special instructions from the prosecutor before testifying.

It should be noted that even the most relaxed of trial judges expects a certain amount of deference from both court personnel and witnesses. A judge's bench or chair is elevated in a courtroom not out of respect for any particular judge but because, traditionally, the judge is symbolic of our respect for the rule of law. Therefore, showing disrespect for a judge becomes translated into a lack of respect for the rule of law and is dealt with severely. Victim witnesses should merely be reminded that the trial judge is neither their advocate nor their adversary; rather, the judge is there to ensure that the trial will be fair and equitable. Given that understanding, the trial judge can usually be relied on to maintain a calm and dispassionate courtroom atmosphere.

Finally, victims should remember that judges, as all people, come in a wide variety of styles, intellect, and personalities; they may be austere, friendly, compassionate, stern, irascible, or even-tempered; on different days, they may perhaps exhibit all of these traits. If the victim is well prepared, it should not matter who the judge is, and the victim should be encouraged to focus her attention and concern on being a prepared and calm witness.

The Role of the Complaining Witness: The Victim

Although much of this chapter has been directed toward the role and conduct of the victim in the courtroom, it might be useful here to discuss some of the more typical questions asked by victims who have decided to testify.

Most victims usually ask how they should dress when they come to court to testify. The simple rule, with some explanation, is to be comfortable and to be natural. Witnesses should wear simple, neat clothing and makeup that is consistent with their age and occupation. There are two major reasons for this rule, one tactical and one practical. The practical reason for dressing comfortably is based on the actual experience of testifying. For many witnesses, the direct examination and the cross-examination may be lengthy. Depending on the jurisdiction, the witness may be expected to sit in a witness box, which is frequently an open, raised platform, or to stand. Obviously, comfortable shoes are a must. Frequently, a witness may be asked to leave the witness stand and walk to a blackboard or a diagram in the courtroom. Short skirts, tight pants, and the like may not only inhibit movement but make the witness self-conscious as well.

The tactical reason that victims/witnesses should dress comfortably and conservatively is because of the continued, although unfortunate, tendency of many jurors to view extremes in clothing or makeup as evidence that the victim was somehow provocative and therefore invited the sexual assault. Many victims are angered, and justifiably so, that it is their lifestyle and not the defendant's conduct that is on trial. The good news is that this attitude is changing, albeit slowly; the bad news is that the victim who wishes to make a political statement by appearing in blue jeans or braless or in revealing clothing will have a more difficult job of convincing the jury that she was raped. The jury has an absolute right, and will be so instructed by the trial judge during the charge, to assess the appearance and demeanor of all witnesses who testify before them and may draw inferences from that appearance in reaching their verdict. Counselors and prosecutors should not hesitate to suggest appropriate attire for individual victims; the defense lawyers will certainly be giving similar advice to their clients.

Many complaining witnesses frequently ask how they should act on the witness stand. Obviously, there is no one answer to this question; victims should be encouraged to be direct and nonevasive. When possible, the witness should attempt to gain, and maintain, eye contact with the jurors since it is axiomatic that people tend to believe those people who, as the saying goes, "look them in the eye."

Theatrics and melodrama should be avoided at all costs. A few years ago, a beautiful young actress who had her first starring role in a play destined for Broadway was sexually assaulted by an armed assailant as she returned to her Boston hotel. Fearing for her life, she complied with his demands. Her assailant was eventually apprehended and, at trial, raised a defense of consent. A jury eventually acquitted the assailant. When questioned following the verdict, a number of the jurors indicated that they simply did not believe the actress because she has recounted the events in a very "theatrical" manner. In a courtroom, especially during a serious criminal trial, every action is magnified because of the solemnity of the environment. It is therefore not only unnecessary but unwise to embellish the facts of the assault; the jury will be far more impressed with a "natural" witness than with one they feel is performing for them.

Many witnesses are afraid, however, that the combination of retelling the incident, along with pointed, if not hostile, questioning from the defense lawyer, will cause them to lose their composure and perhaps even to cry. Although most American adults are extremely embarrassed about crying in public, this potential loss of composure is especially devastating to the victim, who often views it as another aspect of her powerlessness in relation to both her assailant and the subsequent criminal process. If the witness should begin to feel that she is losing her composure to the degree that her personal struggle to avoid crying on the witness stand is interfering with her ability to concentrate on the questions being asked or with her answers to them, she should request a brief recess from the trial judge. The witness should be cautioned that nothing is to be gained by continuing to testify when the judge has offered a recess or her composure is cracking; often the effort necessary to regain control under those circumstances causes the witness to make mistakes and misstatements that could otherwise be avoided.

The witness should also be encouraged to listen attentively to all questions put to her and to answer politely and civilly; perhaps the worst characteristic a victim can exhibit during trial is to appear vindictive in her responses to questions. Moreover, a victim/witness should never engage in an argument with the defense lawyer while she is testifying. She will always lose such arguments because the defense lawyer will know the rules of evidence and at some point will ask the trial judge to instruct the witness simply to answer the questions put to her. Parenthetically, although no less importantly, the emotions generated by such an exchange often cause the victim to lose the concentration necessary to answer any other questions that follow.

Finally, many complaining witnesses are afraid that even with the best of preparation, control, and intentions, they will forget some important detail when they testify. Although for the well-prepared witness this happens very infrequently, several strategies are available. Should the witness find herself unable to remember something, a thankfully rare occurrence, the prosecutor may attempt to refresh her present memory from either the police report, her previous testimony, or her own statement; the witness will not be permitted to read the document to the jury but may read it to herself. When her memory has been refreshed, questions can then be asked of her by the prosecutor. Of course, should the witness totally panic and be unable to testify, even after reading the document, the prosecutor may either request a recess from the judge so that the witness may compose herself or, in certain circumstances, introduce the victim's report into evidence, if it was written at the time of the incident and authenticated by her as representing the facts of the assault at a time when they were fresh in her mind.

Should the witness forget an important detail, the prosecutor may be able gently to prod the witness into remembering by the use of a leading question. Witnesses should remember that leading questions, as such, are not permitted on direct examination and may be excluded on proper objection from defense counsel. However, once again, it is the *question* and not the victim's answer that has been objected to, and the witness, if her memory has been revived by the question, may testify to the forgotten fact in response to another question from the prosecutor. The complaining witness should remember that everyone in the courtroom understands that her role is a difficult one. Should she realize that some part of her present testimony is mistaken or should the cross-examining defense attorney point out some inconsistency with her earlier testimony given at the preliminary hearing or before the grand jury (called a *prior inconsistent statement*), she should attempt to correct her testimony in a nondefensive manner. More harm can be done to the witness's credibility, and therefore to the prosecution of the defendant, by her appearing to be evasive or defensive than in her simply and straight-forwardly admitting the mistake. Perfection is not required, only truthfulness.

A victim who has been direct and specific from the beginning and who has carefully reviewed her original statement to the police, as well as her previous testimony, generally has no difficulty remembering the details of the incident; for many victims, unfortunately, the incident is something which they will never forget. Moreover, there is usually other evidence (hospital records, torn clothing, or fresh complaint witnesses) that will corroborate her testimony. Admittedly, a rape victim must exercise a large measure of self-control while testifying. But, with good preparation, and a modicum of common sense, the experience of testifying need not be as terrifying and humiliating as many victims imagine.

The Role of the Defendant

Up to this point, very little has been said about the role of the defendant. The reason is that, as mentioned in Chapter 7, the burden of going forward and the burden of persuasion that together constitute the burden of proof in a criminal trial remain on the prosecution; the defendant may, if he wishes, remain mute and force the prosecution to prove him guilty beyond a reasonable doubt. What this means, in practice, is that although the defendant's counsel may well cross-examine all the prosecution witnesses, the defendant alone ultimately decides whether or not he wishes to testify or to present any other witnesses in his defense. Even should the defendant decide to present witnesses on his behalf, it must be remembered that he can still choose not to testify.

Since many victims feel that this fact proves that it is the victim, and not the defendant, who is on trial, a brief explanation might be useful. Under our constitutional system, and more specifically the Fifth Amendment to the U.S. Constitution, a defendant has a legal privilege against self-incrimination that is most commonly known as the *right to remain silent*. This right is not peculiar to defendants accused of sexual assault crimes but is extended to everyone who is accused by the government of criminal conduct.[10]

As is true of all constitutional rights, the defendant may waive this right to remain silent, provided that the waiver is voluntarily, knowingly, and intelligently made. Once this is done, usually by the defendant testifying in his own defense, the defendant is subjected to the same rules as any other witnesses. He must testify under oath; he is cross-examined by the prosecutor and subjected to the same tests of credibility as any other witness. The jury may choose to believe or disbelieve his testimony. The important fact to remember, however, is that even if the defendant testifies, the burden of proof does not shift to the defendant to prove that he did not rape the victim. Conceivably, the jury could choose not to believe the defendant's testimony and still find him not guilty if the prosecution fails to prove beyond a reasonable doubt that a crime was committed or that this defendant was the person who committed the crime.

Frequently, victims ask if the defendant will be present when they testify. With the exception of the grand jury, the defendant has the right to be present at all stages of the criminal process. In fact, in the absence of a justifiable excuse, his failure to appear in court either before or during the trial may be introduced against him as evidence of a "consciousness of guilt." Furthermore, the Sixth Amendment to the U.S. Constitution guarantees the defendant not only effective assistance of counsel but also the presence in the courtroom of all persons who can reasonably assist him in his defense.[11] So, unless they are removed by the judge for being unduly disruptive, the defendant, his friends and relatives, and, of course, his lawyer will all be present in the courtroom when the victim testifies.

Depending on the custom in the jurisdiction where the case is being tried, the defendant will either sit in a special box known as the *prisoner's dock* or be seated with his lawyer at a table facing the witness stand. Thus, throughout her testimony, the victim may well find herself looking at the defendant. Again, awareness of this fact should enable the victim to decide how to deal with the situation. Sometimes, defendants will make obvious gestures or show surprise, anger, disbelief, or some other emotion while the

[10]The Constitution of the United States, Amendment V, states in its entirety: "No person shall be held to answer for a capital, or otherwise infamous crime, unless on a presentment or indictment of a Grand Jury, except in cases arising in the land or naval forces, or in the Militia, when in actual service in time of War or public danger; nor shall any person be subject for the same offence to be twice put in jeopardy of life or limb; nor shall be compelled in any criminal case to be a witness against himself, nor be deprived of life, liberty, or property, without due process of law; nor shall private property be taken for public use, without just compensation."

[11]Constitution of the United States, Amendment VI. See text quoted in footnote 3.

victim is testifying. This conduct is improper and, if brought to the judge's attention, will result in an instruction to the defendant to cease all such activity or risk being removed from the courtroom. In any event, the witness should be prepared for the possibility of such conduct on the part of the defendant or his friends and should be instructed to establish eye contact with the prosecutor or the jury regardless of what the defendant is doing. The witness should be reminded that staring down at her lap, if seated, or at her feet, if standing, in an attempt not to look at the defendant may be interpreted by the jury as evasiveness and should be avoided. Some solace for the victim in these circumstances may be found in the fact that most jurors regard such conduct on the defendant's part as inappropriate and unfair and tend to ignore it anyway.

Along the same lines, should the defendant decide to testify, it is equally inappropriate and improper for the victim or anyone associated with her to exhibit the same type of reactions. Unless the victim is able to control her response to what well may be a story diametrically opposed to her testimony, she should be actively discouraged from remaining in the courtroom during the defendant's testimony. Victims should expect that since the defendant's liberty is often at issue, his major purpose in testifying is to present to the jury either a totally different view of the events or to attempt to prove that he was elsewhere when the crime occurred.

The Role of the Jury

Most victims understand that the jury, through its verdict, makes the ultimate decision about the case. Questions frequently arise, however, about the nature of the jurors and their role during the trial. Because the jury does play such an important part in the process, it might be useful to outline how people come to be jurors and what their duties and obligations as jurors are.

Although the procedure varies according to the state where the trial occurs, potential jurors are usually selected at random from the local voting or census lists. Those not exempted by statute (e.g., people in certain occupations) or by personal appeal then form a jury pool or venire.

When a case is called for trial before a judge, a request is sent to the jury pool for a certain number of potential jurors. Those found unfit to serve as jurors in the particular case about to be tried are then excused. Generally, a juror is deemed to be unfit if he or she is related to any of the participants, including the lawyers and the witnesses, or has some other personal or professional interest in the outcome of the case. Both the prosecutor and the defense counsel may then exercise a certain number of peremptory challenges to excuse other potential jurors who they feel would be inappropriate to the case. The 12 jurors plus alternates who are eventually selected (or empaneled) form the petit jury and remain on duty throughout the trial regardless of its duration. The final composition of the petit jury depends on several variables, and the victim should be prepared for the possibility that the final jury may be predominantly male or predominantly female. She should be advised that the sex of the jurors is less important than their individual and collective ability to listen carefully to the evidence and their willingness to reach a verdict based on that evidence.

Immediately preceding the prosecutor's opening statement, the jurors take an oath promising to listen carefully to the evidence and to return an impartial decision, or verdict, based on that evidence. The judge instructs the jurors that they are not to discuss the case with anyone until they begin their deliberations and are not to read or listen to any media stories about the trial. If the judge feels that the case has generated significant media attention, he may choose to sequester the jury by providing them with supervised room and board until the completion of the trial.

Once the trial has begun, jurors are generally not permitted to take any notes or ask any questions of the witnesses or other participants. It is for this reason, among others, that witnesses should speak clearly and slowly. The victim may have reviewed the event hundreds of times in her own mind, but the jury hears the facts for the first and only time when the witness testifies. If the witnesses speak too rapidly or present confusing and disorganized testimony, the jurors may not hear or remember crucial facts. Thus, the best jury will be only as good as the evidence presented to it.

At the conclusion of the judge's charge, the jury retires to a private room to decide on its verdict. A unanimous vote is needed either to convict or to acquit the defendant of the crime charged. Although no specific time limit is placed on the length of time a jury may deliberate, failure to reach a verdict within a reasonable period usually results in a hung jury, and a mistrial is declared. The defendant must then be retried before a different jury at some later time.

The vast majority of jurors view their responsibilities solemnly and earnestly attempt to be fair to both sides, especially in a criminal trial. They realize that the outcome for the defendant is extremely serious; consequently, they regard joking or flippant witnesses negatively, and witnesses should remember this fact when testifying. Finally, witnesses should also remember that these jurors have sisters, mothers, wives, and friends, and to the degree that the victim conducts herself in a reasonable manner, she will have their attention and, frequently, their sympathy.

The Role of the Audience and Spectators

Even those victims who have definitely decided to testify often become extremely nervous and anxious when they are confronted in the courtroom by, as one victim said, "a room full of strangers." Since as a matter of constitutional right the defendant is entitled to a public trial, some attention should be focused on the courtroom audience and what the victim can do to protect her privacy.

Basically, there are three groups of spectators at a criminal trial: (1) disinterested observers, who are frequently students or courthouse regulars; (2) friends and relatives of the defendant and the victim; and (3) representatives of the media.

The first group, while clearly strangers, are often at least initially sympathetic toward the victim, since very few people tend to identify with a defendant in a criminal case. Although students are usually young people, the courthouse regulars are frequently elderly or retired people who attend court practically every day and choose what appear to them to be the most interesting trials. Although these people may be viewed by some as voyeuristic, their presence, once the trial is under way, rarely upsets the witness.

The second group, friends and relatives of the defendant and the victim, obviously have a greater interest in the outcome of the trial. Their presence, although in some respects discretionary with the judge, should be anticipated. Victims should be encouraged to have their own friends and relatives present as long as they are willing to abide by the guidelines previously outlined.

The last group, newspaper, television, and radio reporters, present a more difficult problem to the witness wishing privacy. What occurs in open court during a trial or any pretrial proceeding is a matter of public record and may be reported as such by anyone present; furthermore, the First Amendment to the U.S. Constitution has been interpreted as requiring that the media must not be prohibited from reporting the proceedings in a public trial. The victim should thus be prepared for the possibility that her name and the circumstances of the attack may be repeated outside the courtroom, sometimes in complete and graphic detail. In many jurisdictions, however, rape trials generate little interest among the media unless one of the participants is a public figure.

The rape victim who feels strongly that she will not be able to testify in open court should discuss this with the prosecutor before trial and should request that a motion be made to the judge to exclude spectators during the trial. Even if the prosecutor agrees to present such a motion, there are several considerations to remember. First, the trial judge may refuse to grant the request, either because the defendant objects or because the judge does not believe the exclusion of spectators to be necessary. Second, a closed trial merely excludes the general public. There will still be at least 16 to 20 strangers, including a judge, a court clerk, several (usually at least three) court officers or bailiffs, a court reporter or stenographer, and between 12 and 16 jurors, not to mention the defense lawyer, the defendant, and, in some cases, a defense investigator. Furthermore, as has been noted, the defendant may have any of his friends or relatives present in the courtroom who may be of assistance to him in his defense, *regardless of whether it is a closed trial.* Thus, the victim may succeed in closing the courtroom only to find herself looking at a spectators' section peopled solely by the friends and relatives of the defendant.

Finally, even though the media may be excluded from certain courtroom proceedings, the fact of the trial, as well as the names of the people involved, can still be disclosed. Thus, closing the trial to the general public usually cannot guarantee that it will not be otherwise publicized, unless either the victim or the defendant is a juvenile.

In some jurisdictions, however, such as Massachusetts, legislatures have enacted laws that prohibit "all reports of rape and sexual assault or attempts to commit such offenses and all conversations between police officers and victims of said offenses" from becoming public reports and require that any reports "be maintained by the police departments in a manner which assures their confidentiality."[12] Where such laws exist, criminal penalties of fines and/or imprisonment are usually included in the statute. Although laws of this type cannot guarantee that the victim's name or the circumstances of the assault will not eventually reach the public domain during trial, they usually do allow the victim sufficient time to inform others, if she wishes, about what has occurred and to prepare herself for any resulting publicity.

Whether a trial is open or closed to the public, it is almost always a good idea for the victim to visit the courtroom before the trial begins to familiarize herself with the layout of the room. The general axiom that fear of the unknown is always worse than fear of the known is especially true in the trial of cases involving sexual assault. The well-informed and prepared witness will have far less difficulty testifying and understanding what is happening in the courtroom than the victim who enters uninformed about the process and ill prepared to confront it on its own terms.

---

[12]MGLA, Chapter 41, Section 97D.

IV

Psychological Overview of Rape Trauma

> Crisis is neither an illness nor a pathological experience.
> —Golan (1978)

Rape, like other major life stresses, triggers a crisis response in the victim. This stress does not end when the assailant leaves the scene of the crime. The victim must live with her feelings of helplessness, fear, and vulnerability. Childhood anxieties are frequently aroused by the current distress. With her internal resources already taxed, the victim may find ordinary activities burdensome, and new tasks—like seeking medical attention, working with the police, and deciding how to tell family and friends—may seem overwhelming. Yet it is the mastery of these feelings and tasks that helps to mobilize the victim's strengths, stem her regression, and hasten the process of putting the experience behind her.

A crisis situation may represent a threat, a loss, or a challenge; a threat produces fear and anxiety, a loss incurs depression or mourning, and a challenge stimulates anxiety and hope (Golan, 1978). We believe that there is a combination of all of these elements operating in a rape-related crisis. The specific impact for any given individual is determined by a variety of complex variables. In preparation for offering counseling to rape victims, counselors need to develop a theoretical framework for understanding the psychological impact of sexual assault. We have drawn on crisis theory and psychodynamic formulations to present the reader with a perspective from which to conceptualize rape trauma. This section concentrates on the intrapsychic and emotional responses to rape. It is intended to give the reader greater insight into the psychosocial repercussions and to provide a background for the counseling intervention discussed in Parts V and VI.

Ellen L. Bassuk's chapter sets out the normal, predictable phases a victim goes through in coming to terms with sexual assault. The author reviews crisis theory and the similarities of the response to rape to responses to other crises reported in the literature. She takes a generic approach that focuses on the characteristic course of crisis reactions while allowing for the variations resulting from individual psychodynamics. She goes on to outline the broad issues that she regards as specific to the crisis of rape: the rape work necessary to bring about a resolution.

Malkah T. Notman and Carol C. Nadelson take a psychoanalytic perspective to examine the nature of psychic trauma, with particular attention to the external event as a precipitant. They review the psychoanalytic literature on trauma and emphasize the importance of understanding affects, unconscious fantasies, and ego functions in making an assessment. Their speculations about the affective reactions of guilt, shame, and the inhibition of anger observed in many rape victims is particularly thought-provoking. Adult life-stage developmental issues are discussed in relation to their influence on reactions to rape. In their discussion of the implications for intervention, the authors include indicators for long-term treatment as well as short-term therapy.

Reference

Golan, N. *Treatment in crisis situations.* New York: The Free Press, 1978.

9

A Crisis Theory Perspective on Rape

Ellen L. Bassuk

With the growth of the feminist movement, increasing attention and concern has been focused on the prevalence of the crime of rape and on the nature of the psychological responses of the victim. Rape is no longer viewed as a crime of passion with the victim viewed as complicit but is now seen as a crime of violence inevitably causing an emotional crisis in the life of the assaulted individual. As in other crisis states, such as those precipitated by the death of a loved one or a severe accident or illness, the rape crisis produces a complex set of emotions and symptoms that unfold in a predictable sequence within a specified period of time. Issues unique to the crisis must be resolved and integrated, or the victim will have difficulty returning to her previous level of functioning. The purpose of this chapter is to provide a crisis theory perspective for understanding the spectrum of feelings manifested by the rape victim over the months following the assault. The theme developed is that the crisis response to rape evolves in a predictable sequence similar to other crises, but with a special content specific to rape, which I call the *rape work*.

Review of Crisis Theory Applied to Rape

A crisis is a turning point characterized by a state of intrapsychic disequilibrium in which the individual's usual problem-solving mechanisms are ineffective. The person can neither escape the situation nor solve it by her customary coping skills (Aguilera & Messick, 1974; Brandon, 1970). Sifneos (1960, 1967) defined three factors that must be considered when estimating the severity of a crisis. First, an assessment must be made of the

Ellen L. Bassuk, M.D. ● Assistant Professor of Psychiatry, Harvard Medical School; Director of Psychiatric Emergency Services, Beth Israel Hospital, Boston, Massachusetts.

history of the hazardous situation that is dependent on the degree of the individual's vulnerability. Though it is difficult to imagine a victim who would not be at risk for a crisis reaction to a rape, still one can designate some people who might be more at risk than others. For example, the adult who was sexually abused as a child would be more vulnerable to a severe reaction. The second factor is the nature of the precipitating event. Some rapes involve much more threatened or actual violence than others, some involve much more degradation and abuse than others, and some occur over a longer period of time or involve more than one assailant. Consequently, the severity of the insult itself can vary significantly. The third element is the individual's attempts to resolve the crisis. With rape, one must examine the victim's attempts to cope both during the assault and following her escape from the immediate danger.

In response to a precipitating event that overreaches usual coping mechanisms, the person experiences an increase in anxiety, feels helpless, and develops an array of uncomfortable symptoms. The individual must either change and develop new coping measures or regress. Because the person is in a state of flux, a crisis is an optimal time for effective intervention, which can facilitate not only the individual's resolution of the specific crisis but ultimately support personal growth (Brandon, 1970; Caplan, 1964; Parad, 1965).

An extensive literature exists describing a wide range of crisis situations, such as the birth of a premature child, surgery, physical illness, abortion, divorce, and natural disasters, but the prototype of all crisis responses is the acute grief reaction (Parad, 1965; Rado, 1948; Tyhurst, 1951). Lindemann (1944) first described the grieving process after interviewing survivors and relatives of those killed in the Coconut Grove fire. He described both the characteristic response to loss and distorted, prolonged, or delayed reactions. Central to his description of the natural course of this crisis state is the appearance of acute symptoms and their ultimate successful resolution within a specific temporal framework. During the acute phase, which lasts approximately four to six weeks, five pathognomonic symptoms appear: hostility, guilt, somatic distress, disruption of usual patterns of behavior, and preoccupation with the image of the deceased. Following the acute phase, there is a long process of reorganization during which there is a gradual return to the customary style of functioning. An active process of grieving occurs and then the resolution of the specific grief issues. Lindemann discussed the nature of pathological responses and felt that a population at risk could be identified on the basis of their premorbid or precrisis character styles. He also discussed distorted responses to loss in terms of their deviations from this normal, predictable course.

There is a general consensus among clinicians that the sequence of responses to most crisis situations is similar to that described by Lindemann; more recent work outlines a breakdown of the stages of response to a major stress (Weiss & Payson, 1967; Horowitz, 1976). The anticipatory or *threat phase* consists of the recognition of a potentially hazardous situation. Mounting anxiety serves the purpose of alerting the individual to the risk and mobilizing defenses to deal with the situation or to avoid it. Even when the event cannot be avoided, if the threat phase is long enough it can help to prepare the person by lessening the shock of the experience and allowing for some anticipation of possible coping strategies.

The second stage of a crisis is the *impact phase,* which occurs when the hazardous event cannot be escaped. For rape victims, this phase corresponds to the immediate aftermath of the rape, when recognition of the actual danger is experienced. Victims respond with varying degrees of personality disorganization depending on their character structure and the severity of the trauma. Some victims appear confused, tearful, and shaking; others may appear composed, cool, and without visible affect. In the early days of the impact phase, the victim tries out emergency problem-solving techniques. If unsuccessful, the victim usually feels increasingly helpless and inadequate. The victim may attempt to avoid confronting the impact of the rape by rushing into some new activity, moving, taking a trip, or returning to live with her parents. Others may find themselves preoccupied by the rape. Many women experience flashbacks, intrusive thoughts, or unexpected outbursts of anger or tears. Many cannot concentrate, or they develop phobias, so that routine functioning is impaired. Somatic symptoms such as insomnia, nausea, and gastrointestinal distress are common. The acute symptoms of the impact phase usually last approximately four to six weeks.

The second posttrauma phase, the *recoil phase,* is characterized by a successful implementation of coping mechanisms that result in a decrease of symptoms and a gradual resumption of normal functioning. Although the rape trauma has not yet been resolved, the victim is able to return to her usual level of performance. This early stage of reorganization is managed within the context of an increase in dependency feelings, a limited perspective as to her adequacy and worth, and a need to re-create a supportive interpersonal environment (Brandon, 1970; Tyhurst, 1951). The victim begins to evaluate her ability to cope, which has a major effect on self-esteem and the outcome of the crisis. The presence of an effective support system can provide the necessary reassurance and guidance to facilitate the successful resolution of the crisis. During the recoil phase, victims often seal over their feelings about the rape. As a result, the desire for individual counseling may diminish. Sometimes, a group of other victims can be particularly supportive and comforting, since they provide a forum for sharing a common experience without the intensity of focus of individual counseling.

The later stage of reorganization, or the maximal *reconstitutive phase,* occurs when the victim is able to begin dealing with the specific personal meaning she attaches to the rape. Previously existing conflicts and her life-stage issues play a significant role in determining the individual's concerns. The process of resolving and integrating the rape may take as long as two years if one follows Lindemann's estimate for the completion of the grieving process. The individual emerges with an increase in her adaptive and problem-solving capacity.

The Rape Trauma Syndrome

Within the last decade, because of growing concern about the crime of rape, the media, including prime-time television and radio, have openly confronted women from all strata of society with the possibility of rape. At the same time, a variety of special-interest groups, such as martial arts devotees, have presented their techniques as self-protective. What can be concluded, however, is that there is no prescribed response to an assault and that the highest priority should be the individual's physical safety. Given this mass of information, many women have anticipated how they would respond to an assault and have "tried out" in fantasy a variety of coping mechanisms. Undoubtedly, increased consciousness about the problem of rape has alerted many women to potentially troublesome situations, such as hitchhiking, dangerous urban areas, late hours, and picking up men.

Despite attempts to protect oneself, rape is a crime of violence that is often unavoidable. During a rape, victims experience primal terror and an overwhelming fear of being killed. Symonds (1975) stated that "not only do people submit, but psychological infantilism that occurs with its consequent helplessness makes it appear to the outsider that their behavior was friendly and cooperative. It is a response of frozen fright that confuses everyone."

Once the victim is safe and the external stress is relieved, the victim may express a wide range of feelings, determined in part by her customary coping style. Burgess and Holmstrom (1974) observed the reactions of 92 adult women who were raped and detailed their observations of the rape trauma syndrome. They reported that the victim developed acute somatic symptoms and displayed a wide range of emotional reactions, from numbness and disbelief to hysteria. They categorized the style of response into two groups: controlled and expressed. Although the nature of the reaction is dependent on the individual's developmental stage and character style, most victims described feelings of humiliation, fear, anger, and self-blame.

Notman and Nadelson (1976), in their discussion of the psychodynamics of the rape response, emphasized that feelings of guilt, shame, and anger may be related to unconscious Oedipal wishes that gain expression in universal rape fantasies.

Sutherland and Scherl (1970) studied the reactions to rape of 13 young single women with histories of good prior adjustment. They discussed a three-phase postrape response: an acute period of disorganization with symptom formation and disruption in functioning, followed by a middle phase of denial and repression, and concluded by a resolution phase.

During the resolution stage, the specific rape-related issues must be identified, worked through, and integrated. Despite the fact that victims in this later phase have started to resume their usual mode of functioning, symptoms emerge, such as anxiety and depression, which reflect that the individual is starting to do the necessary rape work. On the basis of six-month follow-ups, Burgess and Holmstrom (1974) have described the following as characteristic: increase in motility manifested by changes in residence, nightmares, and phobias. The nightmares are severe anxiety dreams that probably represent attempts to work through both the manifest and the latent meaning of the rape. Traumatophobia, a symptom discussed by Rado (1948) in reference to the traumatic war neurosis, may also be present in rape victims. In these cases, the victim experiences an increase in anxiety in situations similar to the setting of the assault and therefore tries to avoid any reminder of the rape. Changes of residence may be an attempt to deal with increased anxiety or may be a regressive response, since many young victims return home to their parents for an indefinite length of time. This return home may result in premature closure of the rape-related issues, sometimes preventing their resolution.

Notman and Nadelson (1976) emphasized the importance of viewing the crisis-related issues of rape within the context of the victim's age and life stage, which may determine the nature of these issues. The importance of developmental issues has been popularized in Gail Sheehy's book *Passages* (1974). During each passage, chronological, stage-specific concerns must be confronted and resolved. For example, a late adolescent faced with the task of separating from her parents and defining an adult identity is preoccupied with different issues than the menopausal woman whose children have left home and who is suddenly faced with the loss of her previous role. The adolescent may well be tempted to seek parental protection, giving up her autonomy on the grounds of incompetence. The menopausal woman is more likely to experience the rape in terms of loss of self-esteem and depression, rather than dependency, since her transition from active mothering leaves her vulnerable to questions about her worth and usefulness.

Every victim brings to the rape her own sensitivities and vulnerabilities as they shape her character structure. Horowitz (1976) has emphasized the necessity of understanding the cognitive style of the victim. For example, an obsessional character will demonstrate an exacerbation of the usual obsessional features, and intervention will have to be determined accordingly. This is in contrast to a hysterical style in which there is a preoccupation with emotions and global impressions that are expressed flamboyantly. In addition, preexisting areas of conflict will influence the resolution of the crisis. For example, an individual with a history of early maternal inconsistency and deprivation will bring to the crisis a different set of concerns than the person who has successfully negotiated separation–individuation but had difficulty resolving Oedipal conflicts. The former will suffer a more pervasive sense of self-denigration. She will have more difficulty compartmentalizing the crisis, so that previous functioning will return more slowly. She will struggle with concerns about body integrity and ego boundaries and perhaps develop some serious paranoid fears. On the other hand, the victim who is primarily dealing with Oedipal issues will be better able to contain her feelings, so that there will not be a pervasive disruption of ego functions. She will experience more difficulty in the area of intimate sexual relationships, where guilt, trust, and a sense of worth or desirability may be a problem.

Developmental issues, individual character structure, and preexisting psychopathology are important determinants of the successful outcome of the rape crisis. The specific nature of the issues precipitated by the assault that must be worked through will be colored by these factors.

The Nature of the Rape Work

The Beth Israel Hospital's Rape Crisis Intervention Program has offered medical and psychological care to over 600 victims in the last five years (Bassuk, Savitz, McCombie, et al., 1975; McCombie, Bassuk, Savitz, & Pell, 1976). We have attempted to sort out individual sensitivities and life-stage concerns from more universal issues specific to rape. On the basis of this experience, I would like to suggest that the following three factors are pathognomonic of the crisis response related to rape and comprise the rape work.

1. The victim experiences a breakdown of her usual existential denial of environmental threats. Rape is a crime of violence in which the individual's predominant early response is that she is glad to be alive. However, she has had to confront powerful feelings of vulnerability and helplessness that threaten her basic sense of safety in the world. Usual activities are no longer carried out routinely but are now cautiously reviewed. The victim's freedom to move about safely is significantly curtailed by her extreme sense of vulnerability. She must rework her relationship to the actual space in which the rape took place and to most spaces where there is a threat of assault. Most women limit their degree of freedom in certain geographical areas and

even more extensively at night. The rape victim is even more limited by anxiety and, sometimes, phobic responses. These feelings must be resolved so that the victim is not extensively constricted and then must be reequilibrated with the more ordinary safety precautions or limitations that exist under normal life conditions.

2. The victim experiences a loss of integrity of bodily boundaries because of the rapist's invasion of personal space. This is an important and pervasive theme underlying many issues specific to women and is partly determined by a woman's anatomy and the nature of the sexual act. Depending on the victim's development, she may experience the reawakening of Oedipal issues manifested by guilt and inhibition regarding sexuality. Another victim may experience the rape as a primitive oral threat akin to annihilation, may develop a severe regressive response, and, in the extreme, may become psychotic or suicidal. The victim must rework aspects of her body image and body boundaries, which are intimately connected with self-esteem, before the rape trauma can be fully integrated. She must regain a sense of autonomy over her own body, a sense of reasonable control over her own fate, and a sense of worth and personhood in place of the worthlessness and depersonalization imposed by the rape.

3. The victim must confront the power relations between men and women in our society. Susan Brownmiller (1975) has provided the most extensive and well-documented description of a woman's unequal position before the law. From biblical times, women have been viewed as male property with no rights of their own, including the right to use their own bodies. This position is reflected in common prejudices about rape, such as the belief that women entice their assailants to rape them. During a trial, the defense attorney's cross-examination of the victim about her prior sexual conduct is an attempt to discredit her by suggesting collusion in the crime. On a psychodynamic level, the confrontation of this political reality may reawaken hysterical or masochistic feelings that must be confronted in the rape work. For example, in a hysterical response to the rape trauma, guilt and fear lead to an anxious avoidance of men. In a masochistic response, the fear and anger are turned into self-punishing, self-depriving, or defeatist behavior, as in the case of the student who leaves law school to return to her secretarial job because the rape convinces her that she will never get ahead in a man's world. The rape victim must come to terms with her relationships with the men in her life and rework an altruistic, sharing relationship with her lover or spouse. However, this must be done within the political context of the historical, social, and legal inequities that still exist.

During the long process of reorganization in the rape-related crisis, the victim must confront her feelings in each of the three areas described above. The victim must regain a sense of safety by acknowledging, tolerating, and working through her feelings of vulnerability and helplessness aroused by the assault. She must again learn to feel safe in the space where the rape occurred and master the anxiety of being alone in that space or her freedom will be compromised. The victim must regain a valued sense of self by reworking her sense of body boundaries and integrity. On a more derivative level, this work involves some consolidation of her identity as a worthwhile sexual being and a readjustment of her sexual relationships. This work can be particularly difficult for women vis-a-vis their male sexual partners in a society where women occupy an inferior political power position. Furthermore, these issues must be confronted in the context of any individual pathology precipitated by the assault. In summary, the aim of the rape work is to regain a sense of safety and a valued sense of self and to reestablish sharing, altruistic, mutually satisfying relationships with men in a society where rape remains a threat to all women.

In conclusion, the evolution of the psychological response of the rape victim is similar to the sequence of reactions occurring in other crisis states. What is specific to the rape trauma syndrome is the nature of the rape work that must be accomplished to resolve the crisis. A more complete understanding of these issues can be achieved if systematic research is undertaken for periods longer than six months. Once this research is completed, it will be possible to describe the nature of pathological rape reactions and to formulate guidelines for accomplishing the rape work.

At present, counseling techniques and crisis intervention programs are adapted from models developed for the management of victims of other crises. Understanding the evolution of the rape trauma syndrome and the unique nature of the rape work can lead to the development of programs aimed at the special needs of the rape victim and at the identification of those who are at greater risk of developing longer-term psychological disturbances. Sensitive and timely intervention will lead to more effective management of the crisis of rape and will decrease the psychiatric morbidity for this group of victims.

References

Aguilera, D., & Messick, J. Crisis intervention. St. Louis: C. V. Mosby Company, 1974.

Bassuk, E., Savitz, R., McCombie, S., et al. Organizing a rape crisis program in a general hospital. Journal of the American Medical Women's Association, 1975, 30, 486–490.

Brandon, S. Crisis theory and possibilities of therapeutic intervention. British Journal of Psychiatry, 1970, 117, 627–633.

Brownmiller, S. Against our will: Men, women and rape. New York: Simon & Schuster, 1975.

Burgess, A. W., & Holmstrom, L. L. Rape trauma syndrome. American Journal of Psychiatry, 1974, 131(9), 981–986.

Caplan, G. Principles of preventive psychiatry. New York: Basic Books, 1964.

Horowitz, M. *Stress response syndromes.* New York: Jason Aronson, 1976.

Lindemann, E. Symptomatology and management of acute grief. *American Journal of Psychiatry,* 1944, *101,* 141–148.

McCombie, S., Bassuk, E., Savitz, R., & Pell, S. Development of a medical center rape crisis intervention program. *American Journal of Psychiatry,* 1976, *133*(4), 418–421.

Notman, M., & Nadelson, C. The rape victim: Psychodynamic considerations. *American Journal of Psychiatry,* 1976, *133*(4), 408–412.

Parad, H. (Ed.). *Crisis intervention: Selected readings.* New York: Family Service Association of America, 1965.

Rado, S. Pathodynamics and treatment of traumatic war neuroses (traumatophobia). *Psychosomatic Medicine,* 1948, *4,* 362–368.

Sheehy, G. *Passages.* New York: E. P. Dutton, 1974.

Sifneos, P. A concept of emotional crisis. *Mental Hygiene,* 1960, *44,* 169–180.

Sifneos, P. Two different kinds of psychotherapy of short duration. *American Journal of Psychiatry,* 1967, *123,* 1069–1074.

Sutherland, S., & Scherl, D. Patterns of response among victims of rape. *American Journal of Orthopsychiatry,* 1970, *40,* 503–511.

Symonds, M. The psychological patterns of response of victims to rape. Presented at John Jay College of Criminal Justice and American Academy for Professional Law Enforcement, New York, 1975, pp. 1–18.

Tyhurst, J. S. Individual reactions to community disaster: The natural history of psychiatric phenomena. *American Journal of Psychiatry,* 1951, *107,* 764–769.

Weiss, R. J., & Payson, H. E. Gross stress reaction, I. In A. M. Friedman, & M. I. Kaplan, (Eds.). *Comprehensive textbook of psychiatry.* Baltimore: Williams & Wilkins, 1967, pp. 1027–1031.

10

Psychodynamic and Life-Stage Considerations in the Response to Rape

MALKAH T. NOTMAN AND CAROL C. NADELSON

The experiences that we call rape range from surprise attacks with threats of death or mutilation to insistence on sexual intercourse in a social encounter where sexual contact is unexpected or not agreed upon. Consent is crucial to the definition of rape. The importance of mutual consent is often overlooked and misinterpreted; many people assume that certain social communications imply willingness for a sexual relationship. Although men, women, and children are raped, the majority of rape victims are women; this chapter focuses on understanding rape as a psychological stress for the woman victim.

Burgess and Holmstrom (1974) divided the rape victims they studied into three groups: (1) victims of forcible completed or attempted rape; (2) victims who were "accessories" because of inability to consent; and (3) victims of sexually stressful situations where the encounter went beyond the woman's expectations and ability to exercise control. Despite the different circumstances, the intrapsychic experiences of rape victims in all categories have much in common.

The rape victim usually has had an overwhelmingly frightening experi-

MALKAH T. NOTMAN, M.D. ● Associate Professor of Psychiatry, Harvard Medical School; Liaison Psychiatrist with Obstetrics and Gynecology, Department of Psychiatry, Beth Israel Hospital, Boston, Massachusetts. CAROL C. NADELSON, M.D. ● Professor of Psychiatry, Tufts University School of Medicine; Associate-in-Chief and Director of Training and Education, Department of Psychiatry, Tufts New England Medical Center, Boston, Massachusetts.

Adapted from "Psychoanalytic Considerations of the Response to Rape," *International Review of Psychoanalysis,* 1979, *6,* 97–103; and from "The Rape Victim: Psychodynamic Considerations," *American Journal of Psychiatry,* 1976, *134,* 408–413. Copyright 1976, The American Psychiatric Association. Reprinted by permission.

ence in which she fears for her life and pays for her freedom in the sexual act. Generally, this experience heightens a woman's sense of helplessness, intensifies conflicts about dependence and independence, and generates self-criticism and guilt that devalue her as a person and interferes with trusting relationships, particularly with men. Other important consequences of the situation are difficulty handling anger and aggression and persistent feelings of vulnerability. Each rape victim responds to and integrates the experience differently, depending on her age, her life situation, the circumstances of the rape, her specific personality style, and the responses of those from whom she seeks support.

While rape is basically similar to other crises, its unique feature is contact between two people where one, the victim, is threatened, violated, and subsequently subjected to social condemnation. An appropriate reaction on the part of the victim is not clearly defined. Whether she resists or submits, she feels that she has done wrong. Unlike the soldier who braves an attack in a battle and is praised and decorated, the rape victim is awarded no medal.

For a stress to be psychically traumatic, it must be experienced as overwhelming the ego. In rape, the particular nature of the event and its unexpectedness, as well as the individual's character structure, developmental history, and coping mechanisms, affect her vulnerability. In addition, the event itself may evoke preexisting conscious or unconscious fantasies that contribute to the response. Rape can be viewed as a crisis situation in which a traumatic external force breaks the balance between internal adaptive capacity and the environment. Thus, it is similar to other situations described in the literature on stress, including community disasters (Tyhurst, 1951; Lindemann, 1944); war (Glover, 1941, 1942; Schmideberg, 1942; Rado, 1942); surgical procedures (Deutsch, 1942; Janis, 1958); and other catastrophes.

Psychological Response to Environmental Trauma

The extent and nature of the psychological impact of an external event has been the subject of great interest for many years. Freud (1920) stated, "Such an event as an external trauma is bound to provoke a disturbance on a large scale in the functioning of the organism's energy and to set in motion every possible defensive mechanism." He went on to say that the dreams of those who have experienced severe trauma are attempts at mastery, or that they recover early childhood psychically traumatic memories; thus, they are an exception to his proposition that dreams are wish fulfillments.

The emphasis of psychoanalysis, however, continued to be primarily on neurotic anxiety and was not specifically concerned with external trauma until the more extensive investigations of the war neuroses, in the 1940s. At that time, the consequences of trauma and traumatic neuroses were discussed, and maladaptive responses were reported (Rado, 1942; Kardiner & Spiegel, 1941; Grinker & Spiegel, 1945). Trauma, a concept originally applied to childhood experiences, was extended to include adult stress (Furst, 1967). Mechanisms that are protective against further exposure to trauma but are psychologically costly because they result in loss of self-esteem were described. Kardiner and Spiegel (1941) stated, "as soon as fear is directed inward, in the form of questioning the individual's resources to cope with external danger, or toward the group in the form of questioning its ability to be a protective extension of the individual, then a new and more serious danger situation is created."

Deutsch (1942) and Sutherland and Orbach (1953) observed the impact of illness and surgery. They noted that many of the ill patients they studied were more concerned about the disruption of daily patterns of living than about dying. These reactions were viewed as manifestations of normal adaptation under fear-provoking circumstances, rather than evidence of pathological denial or symptoms of neurotic disorders. Fenichel (1945) pointed to the differences in reactions to external events depending on differences in individual defensive patterns. Greenson (1949) stated that an extreme stress causes the victim to feel helpless, and that the person may resort to extreme defenses, including denial. Identification with the aggressor is also a means of attempting control. Other authors discussed variations in reaction related to sociocultural factors (Wolfenstein, 1957).

Engel (1963) defined the threatening aspects of response to trauma: (1) loss or threat of loss of an object, body part, status, plans, way of life, ideals, etc.; (2) injury or threat of injury, infliction of pain or mutilation that is actual or threatened; and (3) frustration of drives. He pointed out that these categories interrelate and that individual variability is an important factor. Strain and Grossman (1975) have written about the importance of guilt and fear of retaliation, reactivation of separation anxiety, and threat to narcissistic integrity.

Janis (1954), in early work on the subject, stated that the guilt that is often seen is related to aggressive impulses. Thus, a decrease in self-esteem occurs because aggressive impulses are mobilized and experienced by the victim as violations of superego requirements (Deutsch, 1942; Grinker & Spiegel, 1945; Strain & Grossman, 1975).

Furthermore, Janis (1958) stated that threats that cannot be influenced by the individual's own behavior are unconsciously perceived in the same way as childhood threats of parental punishment for bad behavior, resulting in attempts to control anger and aggression in order to ensure that there is no further provocation. This formulation helps to explain the lack of overt expression of anger in so many rape victims and the overwhelming presence of shame and guilt. Janis (1958) also described the exacerbation of neurotic anxiety symptoms that occurs in persons experiencing great stress. Optimistic fantasies about compensatory satisfaction in the future may be used to attenuate anxiety. These fantasies derive from those that functioned as effective reassurances in childhood threat situations. If there is a substantial degree of victimization, however, there is a disappointment in parental figures or those in authority who would be expected to be protective.

In a recent paper, the special developmental influences on the expression of aggression in women has been discussed (Zilbach, Notman, Nadelson, & Miller, 1979). Because there are more stringent restrictions than for men, women have difficulty acknowledging and accepting their own aggression or handling those who agress against them. This fact clearly has special implications for the rape victim.

Those stresses that involve a threat of body damage reactivate early memories of physical danger that have previously been repressed. Past helplessness and lack of control are evoked, and regression occurs (Furst, 1967). Freud (1920) stated that powerful external factors can arouse the weak and helpless child who is submerged under the mask of conventional adult behavior.

Titchener and Kapp (1976) present recent evidence that reactions to catastrophe "are not those of individuals with weak egos" but that the extent of a disaster may reawaken anxieties in most people so that "all of us are susceptible to traumatic neuroses." From their work with survivors of the Buffalo Creek disaster, they also reported that they were able to be effective therapeutically by helping the victims link past and "previously worked through childhood anxieties with the overwhelming anxieties aroused by the disaster."

These descriptions are all applicable to the rape victim, who experiences a threat of death or serious injury, is fearful of retaliation, and feels helpless. She supresses aggression and feels guilty whatever her course of action. This guilt is reinforced by social criticism of her for having been raped, and she is disappointed in people in authority, who often do not support her or give credence to her story.

The preservation or loss of self-esteem is an important component of the reaction to stress. Jacobson (1975) stated,

> Normally, the rise and fall of self-esteem develops in response to actual experiences, such as success or failure, and the intensity and direction corresponds to the nature and extent of the provocation. The more that irrational factors and unconscious conflicts come into play, the more abnormally will self-esteem be altered in its level of intensity and its affective and ideational expression.

She also said that "self-esteem depends on the extent to which the individual can live up to the goals and standards of his ego ideal." In describing responses to war threats, Glover (1941) and Schmideberg (1942) felt that the outstanding mediating factors were the individual's self-attitudes and the loss of previously effective self-assessments that had strengthened that person's sense of invulnerability. Thus, the individual's positive or negative view of his/her ability to cope may change the course of the resolution of that trauma and the future capacity to respond to trauma. A successful response enhances self-esteem; an ineffective one leaves a damaged self-esteem. Since the rape victim is usually blamed for the rape and is sometimes accused of provoking it, she cannot feel successful.

Responses to Rape as a Stress

The profound impact of rape is best understood when it is seen as a violent crime against the person and not as a specifically sexual encounter. Bard and Ellison (1974) emphasized the significance of the personal violation for the rape victim. When an individual is robbed, the robbery is experienced as a violation of the self because home and possessions are symbolic extensions of the self. Stress is intensified when armed robbery occurs because of the coercive deprivation of independence and autonomy, in which the victim surrenders his controls under the threat. When actual injury occurs in a physical assault, there is concrete evidence of the forced surrender of autonomy. Rape is the ultimate violation of the self, short of homicide, with an invasion of the inner and most private space of the individual as well as loss of autonomy and control.

In order to intervene successfully in the rape crisis, one must understand the dynamics of the victim's response to rape. The important considerations in understanding these dynamics are (1) affects, (2) unconscious fantasies, and (3) adaptive and defensive ego styles.

Perhaps most important among the affects is anger. A striking phenomenon in rape victims is the initial display of fear, anxiety, guilt, and shame—but little direct anger. There are several probable reasons for this.

First, since, as indicated above, rape may evoke memories of childhood threats of punishment for misdeeds (Janis, 1958), the victim may feel that she is being punished or is in some way responsible. Her anger may be repressed and experienced as guilt and shame, despite her concomitant feelings of helplessness and vulnerability. Most of the angry feelings appear later in recurrent nightmares, explosive outbursts, and displacement of anger as the woman attempts to master the assault.

Second, expression of aggression in women has been highly conflictual because of cultural restrictions and expectations of passivity and greater compliance in women. Women have often tended toward a masochistic orientation, in which anger is transformed into culturally supported patterns of self-blame. Identification with the aggressor, a mechanism that serves as an attempt to gain mastery, may also make it difficult to acknowledge anger toward the rapist.

Lastly, the socially reinforced suppression of aggression in women has a possible adaptive function, since women are usually smaller and physically weaker than men. Therefore, not responding with a counterattack may prove adaptive. This is an important consideration in understanding the concept of consent. In the past, legal expectations included evidence of force or a struggle in order to establish rape. Current laws accept threat of force as sufficient, recognizing that a woman may submit in fear rather than risk fighting and being overcome.

Guilt and shame are the other dominant affects provoked by rape. Despite the varying circumstances of rape and the different degrees of violence, surprise, and degradation involved, guilt and shame are virtually universal. The tendency to blame the victim, thereby assigning responsibility to her, fosters guilt and prevents her from adequately working through the crisis. It is common for a rape victim to feel that she should have handled the situation differently, regardless of the appropriateness of her actual response. Concerns about the amount of activity or passivity that might have prevented the attack or the rape are frequent. The assumption is that the woman should or could have handled the situation better and that her unconscious wishes perhaps prevented more appropriate assessment and more adaptive behavior.

The guilt of the victim is further increased by focusing on the sexual rather than the violent aspect of the experience. Although aggression is most prominent in the victim's perception, society regards rape as sexual. Since long-standing sexual taboos still persist for many people, even an unwilling participant in a sexual act is accused and depreciated. The popular adage that advises the woman who cannot avoid rape to "relax and enjoy it" misconstrues the attack as a sexual experience. In reality, the rape experience is depersonalizing and dehumanizing. The woman is often a faceless object for the rapist's expression of hostility, and the victim feels degraded and used. Furthermore, since women are expected to exert impulse control in sexual encounters, the rape victim's sense of failure in setting limits, impossible though this may have been, contributes to her guilt.

The question of unconscious wishes translated into the provocation of a rape must be seriously considered. While undoubtedly there are unconscious fantasies in which rape plays a part, and some women do have fantasies in which submission to a stronger man may be linked with forbidden Oedipal wishes, on the conscious level the woman knows that she is submitting because any other behavior would result in real danger to her life. The universality of rape fantasies certainly does not make every woman a willing victim—or every man a rapist. The unconscious fantasy does not picture the actual violence of the experience.

An individual's defensive organization usually protects him/her from acting out such fantasies as may exist. However, if the defensive barrier breaks down and unconscious destructive, aggressive, or masochistic wishes gain expression, anxiety over loss of control combines with guilt regarding the impulses. Rape involves an overwhelming confrontation with another individual's aggression and one's own vulnerability. This confrontation challenges the woman's confidence in her ability to maintain her defenses and controls.

Many women feel some ambivalence toward men as a result of their past developmental experiences. Women expect men to be their protectors and providers, as well as relating to them sexually. Men may also be seen as potential aggressors and exploiters, and the experience of rape confronts the woman with this violent potential. The betrayal by the supposed protector who turns aggressor has a profound effect. Almost all rape victims say that they trust men less after the rape. All men may be suspect, and all are potentially on trial. Uncertainty about one's ability to control the environment reverberates with concerns about the ability to control and care for oneself.

Life-Stage Considerations

It is difficult for anyone to predict how he/she will actually behave in a crisis. In the state of panic evoked during a rape, most women think about how to behave to avoid being physically injured or killed. Some talk, some resist, and others become passive, depending on their assessment of what is going on and their past styles of managing stress (Burgess & Holmstrom, 1976). There are, however, some specific issues related to age and life stage.

The single woman between the ages of 17 and 24 is the most frequently reported rape victim. She is vulnerable often by virtue of being alone and inexperienced. Her relations with men have frequently been limited to the trusted, caring figures of her childhood or the young men she dated in high school. She enters the adult world with little sophistication in some of the nuances of human interaction, and she may easily become involved in an unwelcome sexual encounter. In this age group, the frequency with which rape victims report prior knowledge of the rapist is striking, and this is often the reason for a victim's refusal to prosecute. A young woman may have been raped by a date, an old friend, or even an ex-husband, and she often reproaches herself because she should have "known better" or been more active in preventing the rape.

As was discussed earlier, feelings of shame and guilt are prevalent regardless of the circumstances of the rape; coupled with the victim's sense of vulnerability, these feelings color the victim's future relationship with men. This is especially true for the very young woman who may have had her first sexual experience in the context of violence and degradation.

The experience of rape may revive concerns about separation and independence. A young woman's sense of adequacy is challenged when she asks, "Can I really take care of myself?" Parents, friends, and relatives often respond with an offer to involve themselves in taking care of her again. Although the offers may be supportive and reassuring, they may also foster regression and prevent mastery of the stress and conflict evoked by the experience.

Problems for the younger rape victim also affect her perception and tolerance of the gynecological examination. She may have suffered physical trauma, she is susceptible to venereal disease, and she may become pregnant. An examination is indicated, but it may be perceived, especially by an inexperienced or severely traumatized woman, as another rape. She is concerned about the intactness and integrity of her body and wants reassurance. However, she may have difficulty dealing with the necessary procedures if they stimulate memories of the original rape experience.

The divorced or separated woman is in a particularly difficult position because she is more likely to be blamed and have her credibility questioned. Her lifestyle, morality, and character are frequently questioned. Her apparent sexual availability makes her seem more approachable sexually. She may experience the rape as a confirmation of her feelings of inadequacy, and she is especially likely to feel enormous guilt that can lead to failure to obtain aid or to report the crime. Her ability to function independently is challenged. If she has children, she may worry about her ability to protect and care for them, and others will probably raise questions about her adequacy as a mother. The woman with children must deal with the problem of what, how, and when to tell them about the rape. If the event is known in the community, its implications for her and her children may be difficult to manage.

For the middle-aged married woman, issues of her ability to maintain control and her concerns about independence are particularly important. She is often in a period of critical reassessment of her life role, particularly in the face of changed relationships with her grown-up children. Husbands in their own mid-life crises are often less responsive to and supportive of their wives' sexual and emotional needs.

There is a common misconception that a woman, married or single, who is past her most sexually active period has less to lose than a younger woman. One cannot quantify the self-devaluation and feelings of worthlessness and shame in any woman—especially a woman who may already be concerned about her sexual adequacy.

Implications for Therapeutic Intervention

While keeping the dynamic and life-stage issues in mind, it is important to consider the goals and problems of crisis intervention with the rape victim. The primary goal of a therapeutic intervention in a crisis is a return to the previous level of adaptation and relationship to the social environment. This goal involves understanding and addressing the individual's dynamics and coping patterns, the symbolic significance of the experience, and the life-stage concerns evoked by the trauma. Although the therapeutic principles are similar to those for other types of crisis, particular considerations are related to the specific nature of the rape trauma. Feelings and conflicts about sexuality are aroused because of the sexual aspect of the event. The victim may find it difficult to obtain help because to do so she must reveal herself and reexperience her humiliation. The victim may perceive any medical or psychiatric intervention as equivalent to another rape.

A particularly important aim of therapy for rape victims is to facilitate the reestablishment of a sense of control. Since helplessness, fear, and humiliation are so prominent, the therapeutic encounter must enable the victim to gain and maintain control. It is important to help the victim restore her self-esteem and to support her sense of competence. Regression must be prevented in the immediate posttraumatic period, and, at the same time, therapeutic efforts should be directed toward developing mastery.

Another issue of the immediate crisis period is the effect of the rape on the victim's relationships with significant people. The ability of those in her environment to support her will determine, in part, the extent to which continued therapeutic help becomes necessary. In contrast with most personal crises, where the counselor or therapist reinforces the importance of sharing feelings about the experience with those who are significant in the person's life, no firm guidelines exist about communicating the event of the rape, because of the real possibility that the revelation may disrupt the relationship. Thus, a husband may perceive the rape as a deception by his wife, and the parents of an adolescent may project their own sense of guilt and become angry with the victim. At times, the therapist may have an important role in family counseling. Family and friends must be sensitized to the meaning of the rape so that they are able to give honest support to the victim. Since the rape may intensify preexisting conflicts in relationships, these relationships may be increasingly strained at the very time when the victim needs the most support. If the victim chooses not to tell close friends or family members, guilt or estrangement may occur. If she is able to talk about the experience, mastery is facilitated.

Since the victim feels isolated, alienated, ashamed, and guilty, the initial response to her by professionals, friends, and family is particularly important. Group and family support enables the victim to feel less isolated and helpless. Where possible, the therapist may be helpful in bringing about actual changes in the responses of people to the victim and may help the victim herself to be able to take a more active position. Some victims have sought mastery by helping other victims. The therapist thus has multiple functions and must deal with both intrapsychic issues and environmental realities.

While everyone needs some help in the acute phase, the types of intervention required may differ. In assessing what resources should be offered to rape victims in the acute phase, previous adjustment—including stress tolerance, adaptive resources, and environmental supports—are important to consider. In addition, issues that are specific to life stage must be considered.

Women who have been raped are often reluctant to be labeled as patients, in the usual sense. The idea of being seen as psychologically "sick" may intensify lowered self-esteem. The victim needs reassurance about the way in which she handled the rape and about her efforts to cope following it. She must be offered the opportunity for constructive catharsis with a caring and empathic person.

An additional therapeutic goal, if possible, is to utilize the crisis experience for some further growth. The trauma may be too great for this. However, at times genuine gains may be made. For instance, reactions of significant people may enable the victim to assess her relationships more realistically; the experience may leave her open to intervention and thus to help that reaches to other areas of her life. At times, changes in defensive patterns occur that are more adaptive for the victim than were her previous modes.

It is useful to differentiate short-term crisis goals from long-term issues that require referral for psychotherapy. Those individuals requiring therapy are more likely to be people who have difficulty resolving crises; indications of this difficulty may be a history of deterioration of relationships, phobic reactions, sexual problems, anxiety and depression, or previous instability (of jobs or living situations). In some cases, the nature of the rape itself may have been more traumatic because it involved more violence, because it may have been prolonged, or because it may have been a group rape. It may also have been more closely related to underlying conflicts and previously stressful experiences, or the individual may have been undergoing a concurrent life stress, for example, an impending divorce.

Although crisis-oriented therapy is aimed at restoration of the previous level of functioning, long-term effects of rape also occur and are not always apparent superficially. Long-standing depression or recurrent depressive reactions may follow a rape. The victim may also have difficulty with current and future sexual relationships. She may remain mistrustful of men and conflicted about sexuality. Her sexual partner may respond to her attitude defensively, angrily, or critically, further contributing to the difficulty. Failure in this relationship then accentuates her sense of being helpless, damaged, and incompetent. The therapist can help by predicting and preparing her for these longer-term effects. Counseling for the partner is helpful to enable him to understand his own motivations for his response. Criticizing or blaming the victim and denial of the degree of her distress may be protecting him against awareness of his own vulnerability.

Since, as we know, the tendency to repetition is a response that characterizes reactions to trauma, the rape victim may have recurrent nightmares and phobic responses and reexperience the rape in fantasy. On occasion, some women unconsciously place themselves in a vulnerable position again. This act can be understood, in part, as an attempt to master by repetition. The therapist must be aware of this possibility.

Therapy of the rape victim thus includes the components of short-term crisis-oriented therapy with the additional necessity of working with the impact of the external reality and its implications. The self-esteem of the victim is threatened and likely to be diminished. Shame and guilt related to internalized sexual prohibitions are enhanced by social condemnation and suspicion of the victim, thus making the therapeutic task more difficult. The therapist must be able to see the complex interaction of all of these factors. A focus on one, with consequent neglect of the others, is unlikely to facilitate resolution in a way that promotes long-term gains.

In summary, rape is considered a reaction to a trauma in which the responses are similar to those of other victims of severe stress. The rape response is best understood as the reaction of an unprepared individual to violence rather than to a sexual crime; it is universally experienced as traumatic, evoking previous sexual and aggressive conflicts and reinforced by the real danger and real helplessness of the victim, who remains vulnerable to guilt, problems with self-esteem, and long-lasting impairment in object relationships. Treatment of the rape victim must take into consideration all of these issues as well as external reality and life-stage issues.

References

Bard, M., & Ellison, K. Crisis intervention and investigation of forcible rape. The Police Chief, May 1974.

Burgess, A. W., & Holmstrom, L. L. Rape trauma syndrome. American Journal of Psychiatry, 1974, 131, 981–986.

Burgess, A. W., & Holmstrom, L. L. Coping behavior of the rape victim. American Journal of Psychiatry, 1976, 133, 413–418.

Deutsch, H. Some psychoanalytic observations in surgery. *Psychosomatic Medicine,* 1942, *4,* 105–115.

Engel, G. *Psychological development in health and disease.* Philadelphia: Saunders, 1963.

Fenichel, O. *The psychoanalytic theory of neurosis.* New York: Norton, 1945.

Freud, S. Beyond the pleasure principle. *Standard Edition,* 1920, vol. 18.

Furst, S. S. Psychic trauma: A survey. In S. S. Furst (Ed.), *Psychic trauma.* New York: Basic Books, 1967.

Glover, E. Notes on the psychological effects of war conditions on the civilian population. I: The Munich Crisis. *International Journal of Psycho-Analysis,* 1941, *22,* 132–146.

Glover, E. Notes on the psychological effects of war conditions on the civilian population. III: The Blitz. *International Journal of Psycho-Analysis,* 1942, *23,* 17–37.

Greenson, R. The psychology of apathy. *Psychoanalytic Quarterly,* 1949, *18,* 290–303.

Grinker, R., & Spiegel, J. *Men under stress.* Philadelphia: Blakiston, 1945.

Jacobson, E. The regulation of self-esteem. In E. J. Anthony & T. Benedek (Eds.), *Depression and human existence.* Boston: Little, Brown, 1975.

Janis, I. Problems of theory in the analysis of stress behavior. *Journal of Social Issues,* 1954, *10,* 12–25.

Janis, I. *Psychological stress.* New York: John Wiley & Sons, 1958.

Kardiner, A., & Spiegel, H. *War stress and neurotic illness.* New York: Hocher, 1941.

Lindemann, E. Symptomatology and management of acute grief. *American Journal of Psychiatry,* 1944, *101,* 141–146.

Rado, S. Pathodynamics and treatment of traumatic war neurosis (traumatophobia). *Psychosomatic Medicine,* 1942, *4,* 362–369.

Schmideberg, M. Some observations on individual reactions to air raids. *International Journal of Psycho-Analysis,* 1942, *23,*146–176.

Strain, J., & Grossman, S. *Psychological care of the medically ill.* New York: Appleton, Century, Crofts, 1975.

Sutherland, A., & Orbach, C. Psychological impact of cancer and cancer surgery. II: Depression reaction associated with surgery for cancer. *Cancer Bulletin,* 1953, *6,* 958–962.

Titchener, J., & Kapp, T. Family and character change at Buffalo Creek. *American Journal of Psychiatry,* 1976, *133,* 295–299.

Tyhurst, J. S. Individual reactions to community disaster: The habitual history of psychic phenomena. *American Journal of Psychiatry,* 1951, *107,* 764–769.

Wolfenstein, M. *Disaster glencoe.* New York: The Free Press, 1957.

Zilbach, J., Notman, M., Nadelson, C., & Miller, J. Reconsideration of aggression and self-esteem. (Presented at the Michigan Psychoanalytic Society, April 1979, unpublished.)

V

Psychological Intervention

Skillful psychological intervention immediately following a rape can prevent the development of long-term adjustment problems and strengthen adaptive resources. Counseling may be extremely valuable for those close to the victim as well as for the victim herself.

In Part IV, crisis theory and psychodynamic and developmental considerations were presented to expand our understanding of the trauma for the victim. Part V applies the theoretical material to the actual process of counseling victims and their families and mates. Parts IV and V focus on the intrapsychic and interpersonal experiences of the victim. We assume that the well-prepared counselor will also become familiar with the sociocultural, medical, and legal realities that confront victims and their families.

The reception that the victim receives from those who matter most to her is a decisive factor in how she will view herself and resolve the rape crisis. Counselors must take into account the impact of the rape on the victim's social system and actively elicit the cooperation of family and friends in providing support. This task can be accomplished more effectively when the counselor appreciates that significant others are likely to be in a state of crisis themselves. Helplessness, vulnerability, guilt, shame, and anger are commonly experienced by those close to the victim. In addition, they, like the rest of us, share in the myths and misconceptions about rape and its victims.

In Chapter 11, Sharon L. McCombie and Judith H. Arons present a model for short-term crisis-oriented counseling, adapted to the specific problems and concerns of rape victims. They outline the goals, tasks, and techniques for each phase of the counseling process, which, they point out, must be synchronized with the stages of the victim's reactions to the rape. Two case examples are used to illustrate assessment, treatment, and termination. The authors emphasize that counselors must be alert to the staff stress and countertransference issues that distinguish work with rape victims from other kinds of crisis intervention. They explore the range of feelings aroused in the counselor and discuss how these reactions can potentially jeopardize the counseling process. Their discussion focuses on the female counselor. The stress and countertransference issues for the male counselor are addressed in Chapter 14.

Daniel Silverman and Sharon L. McCombie go on to describe the reactions and concerns of the spouses, boyfriends, and family members of women who have been raped. They discuss the counselor's role as a facilitator for partners and family members to express and understand their own emotions and impulses stimulated by the assault. Family members need to have their personal distress acknowledged and validated. An accepting, nonjudgmental approach is important in making an alliance and promoting adaptive coping measures that are supportive to the victim. With the best of intentions, people close to the victim can inadvertently burden her with behavior that is intrusive or infantilizing. Common defensive reactions to their own distress can lead others to take angry, accusatory stances with the victim or to abandon her emotionally by withdrawing or avoiding feelings associated with the rape. Guidance, modeling, and education about the nature of rape trauma are presented as therapeutic tactics that help to mobilize families to be available to the victim.

11

Counseling Rape Victims

Sharon L. McCombie and Judith H. Arons

Rape victims have undergone an experience of extreme stress that is often sudden, unexpected, and felt to be life-threatening. Our working assumption is that rape arouses massive anxiety that produces a rupture of intrapsychic homeostasis. This in turn precipitates a painful and dysfunctional state of crisis (Golan, 1969, 1978). There are widely observed time-limited and phase-specific emotional and behavioral reactions described as the *rape trauma syndrome* (Burgess & Holmstrom, 1974a,b; Sutherland & Scherl, 1970). Indeed, the rape trauma syndrome is consistent with other gross stress syndromes and crisis reactions reported in the literature (Horowitz, 1976; Lindemann, 1944; Smith, 1978; Titchener & Kapp, 1976).

This chapter discusses a model for counseling derived from this body of crisis theory and from our clinical experience with victims of rape (McCombie, 1976). By necessity, we will be outlining general principles of crisis-oriented counseling. Since this is a summary and overview, we feel that it is important to add two qualifying remarks. First, the clinical research on the immediate and long-range effects of rape on psychological health and growth is still in its developing phase. The clinical observations and theoretical construction used to inform our work with rape victims should not be taken as definitive or conclusive. Rather, we hope to provide a guide that will stimulate thoughtful consideration of the counseling process and that may raise questions for systematic research to expand our knowledge base.

Sharon L. McCombie, M.S.W., A.C.S.W. ● Founder and Director, Rape Crisis Intervention Program, Beth Israel Hospital; Clinical Instructor, Simmons College School of Social Work, Boston, Massachusetts. Judith H. Arons, M.S.W., A.C.S.W. ● Staff Social Worker, Obstetrics and Gynecology Service, Ambulatory Care Unit, Beth Israel Hospital; Clinical Instructor, Simmons College School of Social Work, Boston, Massachusetts.

Second, our purpose is to develop a counseling model that reflects the individual and intrapsychic context in which a rape is experienced. We are aware of the danger of too narrow a point of view. An exclusively psychological orientation runs the risk of ignoring the larger social and political issues surrounding rape, while a purely political approach loses sight of the individual victim's personal response. Those who view rape primarily as a political issue charge that the intrapsychic approach casts further blame on the victim. On the contrary, we believe that the exploration of the idiosyncratic meaning that rape carries for the victim and the clarification of feelings of complicity and guilt are central to the process of gaining a realistic perspective on the assault. We also believe, however, that counselors must educate themselves about the sociopolitical conditions that perpetuate rape (Brownmiller, 1975).

The assessment and treatment of rape victims does not differ substantially from the process of counseling people in other kinds of acute distress. However, because rape is a highly charged issue surrounded by powerful myths, the counselor must be prepared to examine and deal with her feelings about rape in general and to disabuse herself of the stereotypes and misconceptions she might hold. In addition, counselors must expect to be stressed by hearing about assault situations and the victims' feelings of helplessness and fear in the face of an overwhelming reality. Similar feelings are elicited in the counselor. One study of counselors in a rape crisis intervention center found that they experienced some of the stress symptoms of the rape trauma syndrome (Zonderman, 1975). The emotional exhaustion that results from crisis intervention can produce a gradual erosion of caring and commitment: staff burnout. It is important that staff stress be expected, acknowledged, and compensated for by support measures such as staff training, clinical supervision, case discussions, and diversification of tasks and case load.

Staff Stress and Countertransference

Because staff stress is so prevalent in rape crisis counseling, we will review some of the major difficulties inherent in listening to accounts of rape. During the treatment process, the counselor is forced to confront in herself feelings that mirror what victims experience: vulnerability, helplessness, rage, guilt, shame, and fear. These emotions are anxiety-provoking and may be defended against by methods that can interfere with the counselor's capacity to be helpful to the victim. The therapeutic task with rape victims is the same as with any trauma victim: to provide sufficient containment of powerful affects within the counseling relationship to enable the client to remember, reexperience, understand, and come to terms with the assault. For the rape counselor, this means a confrontation with both her own personal vulnerability to danger and her own masochistic and sadistic feelings.

We all live with considerable existential denial of the risks in our environment. None of us likes to consider the fragility of our lives or to think about the risks we take on a daily basis, like driving a car, taking a plane, or smoking a cigarette. We all rely to some degree on omnipotent fantasies to shelter us from experiencing our mortality so immediately. Hearing stories of women who have been attacked and raped in the course of doing ordinary things forces an abrupt realization of our own vulnerability. We may find ourselves fearful about walking to the parking lot and anxiously checking locks on windows and doors once we get home. The world is no longer such a safe or predictable place; we begin to look over our shoulders and startle at unexpected noises.

In order to protect herself from this kind of discomfort, the counselor may unconsciously resort to blaming the victim as a way of distancing herself from the fear that "It could have been me." Particularly in cases where the victim may have shown poor judgment in her behavior, such as hitchhiking or riding home from a party with a stranger, the counselor may focus on this behavior as the *cause* of the rape. That is, since the victim opted to put herself in a risky situation, the rape that ensued must have been her "fault." This kind of retrospective critique is often in the service of supporting the counselor's need to maintain her view of herself as the mistress of her fate. By locating the "mistake" made by the victim, the counselor is reassuring herself that *she* would never do anything like that; therefore, she is safe. Especially in instances where the victim's judgment was poor, the counselor needs to align herself with the victim's observing ego, in order to explore what may have contributed to her lack of sound judgment. For this to be accomplished, both victim and counselor must get beyond the casting of blame and harsh judgments to achieve a realistic appraisal of the victim's motives and behavior. This task cannot be accomplished if the counselor is unconsciously involved in condemning the victim in order to protect her own need to feel in control.

The counselor's masochistic and sadistic feelings can easily be tapped by the victim's descriptions of brutality, subjugation, and suffering. For example, hearing about a rape, especially when perversions or vicious brutality are reported, can be experienced by the counselor as a kind of secondary assault. Bearing the shared horror of the rape can make the counselor feel victimized herself. In other words, she becomes identified with the victim's masochistic position, and particularly so if she and the victim are of a similar age and background. Such an identification threatens to make conscious the counselor's censored masochistic fantasies, and she may respond defensively in disgust or fear.

On the other hand, listening to rape accounts may provoke an outburst of the counselor's sadistic feelings. It is commonplace for counselors to remark on their wishes to "kill that bastard," to castrate him, or to torture him so that he will get a taste of his own medicine. Such intense rage reactions arouse considerable anxiety in the counselor, particularly if she has a high investment in viewing herself as compassionate and caring. She may feel ashamed and guilty about such thoughts, or superego injunctions may lead her to repress these feelings altogether. The counselor's anxiety about her own aggression and sadism can make it very difficult to be attentive and tolerant when the *victim* brings up her own sadistic response to the assailant. The victim's anxiety about losing control of her aggression is commonly present, although it may be defended against by projecting such impulses onto an irate husband or by excessive concern for the "poor sick man" who raped her. In fact, sometimes the phobic behavior of the victim who does not leave her house for fear of a repeated assault involves an unconscious wish to go out and murder her assailant. The guilt and sense of wrongdoing verbalized by many victims can sometimes be traced to the internal aggression and sadistic fantasies evoked by the violence suffered.

Rape is a prototypical symbol of sadomasochism, and indeed, work with the victim has certain countertransference issues in common with work with assailants or those who have committed sadistic acts (Haley, 1974). Both situations compel the counselor to face the horror of actual sadistic behavior and the reality of human beings committing violence against one another. In order to maintain the necessary empathic alliance with her client, the counselor must recognize and tolerate her own impulses to be violent, as well as her own potential to be an object of violence. If she does not, the counselor will eventually either blame and reject the victim or collude with her to avoid discussion of these very distressing and unsettling subjects.

Counselors also frequently report feeling uncomfortable about asking for explicit details of the rape. They worry about being voyeuristic and intrusive in asking to hear exactly what took place. Sometimes, the counselor may find herself confused about her motivation and feel both fascinated and repelled by the details, or she may be titillated as the victim talks about various sexual acts. These feelings evoke shame and guilt in the counselor. In order to protect herself from feeling uncomfortable, the counselor may avoid asking for this information. Inadvertently, this avoidance can give the victim the message that her experience is too shameful to be discussed. Since victims are struggling with their own guilt and shame about the sexual acts, it is very important to provide the opportunity to share this part of the experience as well.

In order to understand the mutual discomfort that counselor and victim feel about the details of a rape, we need to remember that we are all trying to master fears, prohibitions, and confusion stemming from our conflicts about sexual and aggressive feelings. A report of rape catalyzes anxieties related to our own conflicts. While this chapter cannot do justice to the various permutations these issues can take in the countertransference of counselors, we do believe one much-referred-to phenomenon bears some discussion: women's rape fantasies.

Most of us at one time or another have had them. They may be in the form of erotic dreams or waking thoughts accompanying masturbation or intercourse. The imagined scenario produces excitement and sexy feelings. These fantasies function both to gratify our sexual desires and to mollify guilt about such wishes by removing responsibility for these feelings. It is as if the rape fantasy is a way of saying, "I was just minding my own business when this handsome sheik scooped me up on his horse and abducted me to his tent and insisted he must have me—what could I do?" Such fantasies are pleasurable and the rape is nonviolent.

Sometimes rape fantasies take the form of a frightening nightmare in which the erotic component is slight and the overriding focus is the hostility and violence. Such nightmares may be expressing the fear of punishment for sexuality: loss of control, humiliation, destruction. Sex is unconsciously experienced as dangerous and forbidden; to indulge is to risk terrible retribution. Such nightmares may be expressions of the hostility and aggression of the dreamer, projected onto and displayed by the attacker. The sadism of the rapist symbolizes the dreamer's sadistic feelings, but because of superego prohibitions against such impulses, they are played out by another character in the dream.

Regardless of whether the rape fantasy is predominantly associated with sexual or aggressive feelings, it is an expression of conflict. It is also an internal activity that neither arouses nor hurts anyone else. The fantasizer is the writer, producer, and casting director of her own private dream script, be it X-rated or scary. Meanwhile, she is safe in her bed. Being raped in reality, however, is not safe and not sexy.

The prevalence of rape fantasies in women is sometimes cited as proof that all women secretly desire to be raped, and it is used to deflect responsibility for actual rapes away from the rapist. Women want sexual pleasure, and fantasizing about rape can be sexy. Being raped in fact is literally to be forced to have sex when one does not want to have sex. Thoughts or fantasies about murdering or being murdered are also common. To argue that a person wanted to be killed because he had a fantasy of being murdered is hardly a justification for a killing. If we were all held accountable for our wishes and thoughts, most of us would be behind bars.

Rape fantasies can be a source of shame and guilt in both counselor and victim. It is difficult to reconcile the pleasure associated with most rape fantasies with the pain experienced during an actual rape. When an event corresponds to a fantasy, we can lose sight of the boundary between fantasy and reality or slip into magical thinking about a causal relationship. The actual rape may then be experienced by the victim as punishment for her fantasized rape. For the counselor, hearing about a rape may arouse associations about her own rape fantasies and result in anxiety and guilt.

When the counselor is alert to the possibility of such reactions, she is able to control acting on these feelings. If the responses are unconscious, the counselor may behave in ways that are destructive to the therapeutic task. All of us have an aversion to recognizing malicious or masochistic tendencies in ourselves, since they are inconsistent with maintenance of our self-esteem. All of us have some guilt and anxiety about our sexual impulses. For the most part, these feelings are repressed. The stimulation of listening to rape accounts threatens that repression. The counselor must be prepared to encounter and take responsibility for her feelings and conflicts. Awareness of the stress and the countertransference reactions is necessary to forestall behavior that is harmful to the counseling process and to the victim.

The Counseling Process

The counseling model presented in this chapter is short-term (usually 12 sessions or less) and is directed toward restoring the victim to her precrisis level of functioning. If a victim's baseline functioning is seriously impaired, then this model may not be appropriate. As with any random sample of the population, rape victims range anywhere along the spectrum of emotional health and illness. Clearly, if the victim is psychotic, borderline, or suicidal, the clinician must gear her intervention accordingly. For example, medication, structure, reality testing, and mobilization of family and community resources may be the bulk of the acute work, with referral for longer-term treatment or hospitalization for follow-up.

When counseling is initiated within the first few days following a rape, the victim is likely to be in the first phase of the rape trauma syndrome. She may appear somewhat dazed and may describe a sense of unreality about the rape as she struggles to comprehend what happened to her. She may be visibly upset, crying, and trembling and may have trouble communicating in a coherent or logical fashion. Or she may appear calm and composed and may articulately state, with little overt sign of distress, exactly what took place. In other words, there is a wide spectrum of how victims may present following a sexual assault.

To some extent, elements in the assault will influence the degree of stress. These include the amount of violence, her prior relationship with the assailant, and the extent of the injuries sustained. The presence of concurrent stresses in the victim's life will also effect her ability to manage the rape sequelae. For example, has there been a recent breakup with a boyfriend, or a shift to a new job, or a death in the family? The responses of family, friends, and institutions to the news of the rape will increase or decrease stress. Were the police respectful and helpful? Did her parents get angry with her for walking at that time of night? Finally, the individual victim's character structure, her ego functions, and her usual problem-solving patterns are most significant in determining the quality and quantity of the traumatic impact.

During the first days and weeks following the rape, the victim contends with decisions about medical care, police involvement, and physical security precautions as well as whether and how to tell family and friends about the assault. Still reverberating to the loss of control, helplessness, and fear evoked during the rape, the victim is likely to feel tense, preoccupied, and exhausted and to have difficulty concentrating and performing her routine tasks. Symptoms appear as emergency methods to bind the anxiety that threatens further disorganization. These include sleep disturbances, nightmares, changes in appetite, intrusive thoughts, phobias, startle reactions, increased suspiciousness, diffuse anxiety, and depression. Victims report loss of interest and/or apprehension about sex. Physical complaints unexplained by direct injury, such as headaches, gastrointestinal discomfort, and aches and pains may occur, particularly in people who tend to somatize. These changes in personality, mood, and functioning during the first weeks following the rape cause many victims increased anxiety, since they then feel out of control of themselves. They may worry that they will never be the same or, in the extreme, that they are "going crazy."

The goal of counseling during the acute aftermath of the rape is to help the victim to organize herself. She needs to begin to acknowledge and comprehend the impact of the rape and to give herself permission for a time of healing without harsh self-criticism or unrealistic expectations. She needs to begin to reestablish confidence that she can take care of herself by identifying what she needs to do now and by taking steps to mobilize herself to accomplish her goals. In the initial phase, the counselor's job is to establish an alliance with the victim; to determine her major concerns; to formulate an assessment of her coping strengths; to evaluate the meaning and impact of the rape in terms of her personality structure, developmental life-stage, and preexisting conflicts; and to make an agreement with her about the focus of the counseling.

The crisis nature of the counseling requires that the clinician be flexible and active in her approach. Because of the pressure to make a rapid assessment and elicit the necessary relevant information to do so, the initial interview is usually the most anxiety-provoking for the counselor. Depending on the needs of the victim, the counselor may decide to structure the interview or to keep it more open-ended to facilitate the ventilation of feelings and concerns. For example, if a victim is very upset, volatile, and confused, the counselor will provide an organizing framework by offering reassurance to calm the victim and questions that begin to help the victim to organize her thinking. If the victim is composed, the counselor may choose more open-ended questions to elicit her affective experience.

Generally, the counselor must respect the victim's need for a nonjudgmental, noncontrolling interviewer. It is imperative that the counselor identify and support the victim's ego strengths and not encourage regression. Since the victim is still raw from an experience of having lost control, it is critical that the counselor work toward moving the client to an active and mastery-oriented position. One pitfall for counselors is that in their zeal to be helpful and reassuring, they may inadvertently infantilize the victim by telling her what to do or by doing things for her. Unwittingly, passivity and dependence are elicited, and the victim's worries about her capability to manage as an effective adult are reinforced.

Making a psychosocial assessment of the victim in the acute phase is difficult. Because of the regression produced in the immediate aftermath of the trauma, the victim's ego functioning is taxed, and consequently, ego deficits and more primitive defenses are pronounced. Furthermore, the victim is likely to be too preoccupied with the rape itself and its repercussions to find discussion of her past useful or relevant. While in most other counseling situations, the client expects to reveal personal issues, the victim's recent violation may make her extremely sensitive to further exposure. Thus, the historical material necessary to assess baseline functioning comes slowly or in a piecemeal fashion, often making it difficult during the first interview to assess the degree of the victim's regression.

We will outline the main tasks and techniques that counselors should find useful throughout the stages of rape crisis counseling. In order to clarify the outline, we will introduce two victims, Sally T. and Barbara D. This clinical material should break down the artificial boundaries used in laying out a theoretical framework. Sally T. is a young woman with many internal strengths and a satisfying career and social life. For her, the rape was a relatively contained situational disturbance. On the other hand, Barbara D. is a young woman with a history of poor self-esteem, depression, and highly conflictual relationships. For her, the rape is one of many problems, and it has highlighted preexisting deficits. One of the most frequent dilemmas for crisis counselors is how to accomplish a focused and contained piece of work, particularly when long-standing conflicts are in evidence. We describe Barbara D. in more detail below and use her treatment to illustrate the goals and techniques presented in the following outline. At the end of each section, excerpts from Sally T.'s therapy are introduced to provide more of the flavor of the overall treatment process.

Barbara D. is a 19-year-old college freshman at a large urban university. She grew up in a small town in Vermont with her mother, father, and older sister. Barbara had moved to the city to attend college only two months before the rape. Her assailant was a young man she had met at school a few weeks earlier. Barbara explained that on their first date, he asked if they could stop by his room to pick up his wallet. Once there, they had a drink and began to talk. They kissed a few times, but Barbara rebuffed his attempts to touch her breasts. At this point, they resumed their conversation, and the young man began to discuss his childhood and how angry he was at his father. Barbara reported that her date then "became wild" and began to slap her face. He threw her down on the floor, took off her clothes, and forced her to have oral sex and vaginal intercourse. During the assault, he said that he "loved" her and wanted to "make a woman" of her. Barbara described feeling unable to move or to make a sound. She felt that if she didn't cooperate, she might be killed. The episode lasted about an hour, after which he apologized to her and sent her home in a cab. Barbara had been a virgin until this time.

Once back at the dorm, Barbara showered and cried herself to sleep. It wasn't until the next morning that she told a close friend and called her mother. With her friend's support, Barbara came to the emergency room. The staff described her as "quiet and shy" and "unable to make eye contact." She had a pelvic exam, was treated prophylactically for venereal disease, and was informed about what legal steps she could take if she chose. Barbara did not report the assault to the police but did agree to speak with a counselor. They contracted to meet for 12 sessions.

I. *Initial Phase of Counseling*
   A. Tasks
      1. *Initiate a supportive relationship.* Provide the victim with reassurance about her physical safety and personal integrity and encourage an alliance through empathic listening and communicating understanding of the victim's pain.
      2. *Identify the victim's major concerns and her perception of the kind of help she needs.* Are her worries mainly about her own reactions and future adjustment (psychological intactness: overt counseling request)? Does she focus on concerns about venereal disease or pregnancy (physical intactness: overt medical request)? Is she preoccupied with the apprehension of the assailant (retribution: overt police–legal assistance request)?
      3. *Educate about medical care, police investigation, and court procedures.* This reduces anxiety about the unknown and supplies the data necessary for the victim to make informed decisions.
      4. *Mobilize the victim to use the social supports available to her.* If she anticipates blame or rejection, reality-test these worries. Offer to meet with family and friends to provide guidance and education and to assess their need for further counseling. Evaluate the accessibility and effectiveness of her social network.

5. *Anticipate with the victim what feelings, thoughts, and symptoms that she might experience in the immediate future.*
6. *Encourage the victim to make plans for her safety and support for the next few days.* If necessary, make referrals for medical care, alternative shelter, child care, advocacy for police–legal concerns, etc.
7. *Make an agreement with the victim about the counseling contract.* This includes a tentative formulation of the focus, a clarification of the counselor's role, and an approximation of frequency and duration of visits.
8. *Begin to make a psychosocial assessment with particular attention to ego functions.*
   a. Elicit feelings and observe appropriateness, intensity, lability, and mode of expression of affects. Be alert for feelings of complicity, irrational guilt, anger, and shame. Note the amount of anxiety present.
   b. Assess defensive structure. What are the major defenses used, how rigid/flexible are they? How adaptive/regressive are they?

For example, in the first few interviews, Barbara D. was unable to discuss the sexual aspects of the assault. She handled her anxiety and shame about them by suppressing her feelings and by a flight into activity at school. She became obsessed with schoolwork in an attempt to displace anxiety from the rape onto a less threatening area of her life. This obsessional defense was successful during the first few weeks after the assault. It enabled her to continue functioning autonomously in an area that was vital to her self-esteem. But by the fourth interview, Barbara was openly discussing her guilt (she felt she was "bad" to have gone to the assailant's room), and thoughts about the rape disrupted her concentration at school. Barbara then began to feel the depression and anxiety that had threatened to disorganize her after the assault, but she could now tolerate them without any major disruption in her functioning. Although Barbara later revealed evidence of significant pathology, her original displacement, avoidance, and obsessional maneuvers were initially very adaptive. Giving up these defenses and moving toward increased affect tolerance pointed to an important personal strength.

   c. Assess the nature and degree of symptom formation, particularly the extent of dysfunction that results. For example, the victim may have difficulty falling asleep but is still getting adequate rest. If the sleeplessness increases or lasts beyond the first week, a sleeping medication might be prescribed. The victim may be fearful about going out alone after dark, but this fear only minimally restricts her work and social life. On the other hand, the victim who refuses to leave her house at all has a phobia that significantly compromises her functioning.
   d. Look at her coping and problem-solving style, including her help-seeking behavior. How did she react during the assault? For example, did she attempt to negotiate some control by bargaining with the assailant? Did she dissociate and feel apart from what was happening to her body? Did she resign herself to the rape and become passive, or did she physically struggle or scream? Can the victim take satisfaction in the way she handled the assault, or is she critical of herself? What did she do immediately following the rape? Whom did she contact and why?

In the case of Barbara D., feelings of guilt and shame initially interfered with her ability to get help, and although she was quick to engage with the counselor, many women who feel deeply ashamed require more active outreach. Rather than telling a close friend or relative or immediately getting medical attention, Barbara went to her dorm and spent the entire night alone. During the first few interviews, she appeared to be preoccupied with her compliance during the rape, and for several weeks, she remained extremely critical of her behavior during the assault. This preoccupation was a clue to the counselor that the rape was probably exacerbating prior conflicts about passivity, sexuality, and possibly masochism.

> e. Determine the quality of her relationships and her capacity to use them for support. Are they mutually satisfying or exploitative, growth-promoting or regressive, superficial or substantial? Does she anticipate that she will withdraw from others, or will she be able to seek support? Is she concerned that she will lose the respect of others as a result of the rape or, in the extreme, that she will be rejected? Does she anticipate that she will end up taking care of others (like a distraught mother or an angry, impulsive boyfriend)? Can she tolerate the concern and assistance of others, or will she be help-rejecting?
> f. Ascertain a general sense of her baseline functioning.

For example, in the first interview, the counselor noted that prior to the assault, Barbara D. had been functioning as an average college student, had left home, and had made an important friendship with another young woman. She had no previous psychiatric contacts or hospitalizations and no history of drug abuse or delinquency. This information gave the counselor some sense of Barbara's usual capabilities and helped her in considering what treatment goals would be realistic.

> g. Ask for a crisis history. Look particularly for losses, major illness, accidents, abortions, and assaults. How did she react then, and what worked or didn't work for her? Does she relate the rape to any other time of crisis in her life, and if so, how? This information is useful in helping the victim to anticipate her own reactions, thereby increasing her self-control.

For example, in the second interview, Barbara D. revealed that she had experienced a number of family crises while growing up in Vermont. Her father was an alcoholic prone to unpredictable displays of violence. Barbara recalled one particular episode in which he lunged for her without warning and threw her to the floor. She reported the same feeling of paralysis and helplessness that she had experienced during the rape. As she spoke of her past, Barbara related the rape more and more to her experiences with her unpredictable father. The counselor helped her to anticipate that she might feel the same depression that had followed these earlier incidents at home.

> h. Consider general life-stage issues and how the rape may make an impact on developmental tasks. For example, if the victim is in her 60s, dealing with failing health and anticipating retirement, the rape may be experienced as confirmation

of her diminishing strength and status. She may become depressed and preoccupied with death and isolate herself from family and friends.

At the other extreme, Barbara D.'s rape coincided with her attempts to master the tasks of late adolescence: separation from family, choice of a nonincestuous love-object, and consolidation of career or work plans. Occurring at this time in her life, the rape threatened to undermine her autonomous functioning and exacerbated unresolved conflicts around dependency and sexuality.

B. Techniques
1. *Concentrate on the affective experience of the here and now.* The victim should be encouraged to put her feelings into words in order for her to gain some sense of self-control. The counselor can label amorphous feelings in order to facilitate this articulation. For example, the victim may say that she doesn't know what she's feeling but that all she can think of is the image of his hand holding the knife. The counselor might remark, "Sounds like you're very scared about how close you came to being killed."
2. *Maintain a calm, attentive, and concerned demeanor.* This is reassuring to the victim and conveys the silent message that she will not be rejected. It is important to help her to realize that while the assault is unacceptable behavior, *she* is not unacceptable.
3. *Avoid being controlling, since that approach will create a resurgence of her feelings of helplessness and the need to ward off further intrusiveness.* If the victim is silent, ask, "Is it OK if I just sit with you for a while?" This silence gives the counselor time to consider why the victim is so quiet. Is she dazed, or overwhelmed by feelings, or mistrustful of others? Nonverbal demonstrations of concern can be helpful, such as bringing her coffee or tissues. The counselor might ask, "What can I do to help you feel more comfortable?" Empathic statements that do not challenge the victim or require her to respond are useful in conveying understanding. For example, "You must be exhausted and drained right now."
4. *Ask general questions and move gradually to more specific inquiries.* This process allows the victim time to become familiar with the counselor and to develop a rapport before more anxiety-provoking material is approached. For example, the counselor may ask whether she works or goes to school, then proceed to where she was and what she was doing when she first sensed that she was in danger.
5. *Use clarifications, labeling, generalizations, and reflections to facilitate communication and convey understanding.* For example, "Many women who have been raped are worried that they should have somehow been able to prevent the rape. Is that a concern of yours?" Or when Barbara D. explained that she hadn't told anyone about the rape until the next day, the counselor clarified the meaning of this behavior by responding, "Perhaps it was hard to tell someone because you felt partly responsible for the rape and feared that others might blame you for what happened."
6. *Support existing adaptive defenses.*
7. *Deal with affective concerns as they are raised by the victim.* It is important to let the *victim* establish the emotional tone of the interview. Attempts to push for a catharsis will undermine her coping skills and cause further regression or decompensation. On the other hand, avoidance of feelings can play into the victim's depressive response to the assault (that she is bad, unworthy) or confirm her anxiety that no one can understand or help her tolerate her feelings.

8. *Underscore the options she has open to her as a way of encouraging her to take an active role in her recovery.* This approach also conveys a sense of hope that things can and will feel different. By circumscribing and ordering priorities, the victim will feel in a better position to manage.

Case Example: Sally T.

Sally T. called our rape crisis intervention program two days after she was raped. She reported that she had sought medical care and had gone to the police and that she was now staying with friends. She wished to make an appointment to speak with a counselor. She was having trouble sleeping, had lost her appetite, and found herself extremely anxious and jumping at the slightest provocation. Her friends were very supportive and were telling her how well she was doing. She agreed that she was taking appropriate steps but that inside she felt shaky. An appointment was made for the following morning.

Sally T. presented as a 25-year-old single nurse who lived alone in Boston. She was a small, tomboyish woman, who was very articulate and composed. In a calm and matter-of-fact fashion, she began the interview by recounting the incident and her reactions during the first 72 hours following the assault.

In brief, she had been getting ready for bed after returning from dinner at a friend's house. She was startled by a man standing in the doorway of her bedroom. He was an orderly from the hospital whom she knew slightly and who lived in her neighborhood. He did not have any weapon, but he was a large, heavyset man. He had been drinking and was "acting crazy," very much unlike his usual low-keyed manner. Sally said she was scared but tried to keep calm and to talk to him. He became increasingly agitated. He forced Sally to perform fellatio on him and to have intercourse. He then became calm and polite and left the house. Sally said that she was dazed as she went around the house making sure all the locks were fastened. She discovered that the back door had been jimmied. She called her best friend in New York City, who advised her to call a local friend, which she did. This friend brought her to her apartment, where Sally alternated between crying and feeling a sense of disbelief. She vomited and finally slept fitfully for a few hours. That morning, she called the police, who took her to a hospital. The man was arrested the following day.

Sally discussed how confused and worried she felt about pressing charges. She repeatedly said how disturbed the man was and how badly he needed help. She saw the rape as a plea for intervention: "He knew I would call the police. He knew he'd be caught." When he was released on bail, she was very upset because "He's not getting any help. He may get more desperate and do something again." Her concern that the man get psychiatric care was her major preoccupation in the first interview.

The counselor asked what concerns she had for herself. Sally said that she was worried about how the rape would effect her future relationships. When asked if she was concerned about men specifically, she said, "No, both men and women I guess. It's just that I knew him. He seemed like a quiet, nice guy. I'm worried I'll never trust anyone again." The counselor inquired if this worry was effecting how she felt with her friends: "Well, not exactly. My friends are being wonderful. But it's hard for me to let them take care of me. I'm not used to it. I've always been very independent, and I don't like feeling needy. Since the night of the rape, I haven't felt much except anxious."

The counselor inquired if she had ever noticed this reaction in herself before. Had there been any other time of upset? Sally reported that she had had an abortion six years ago. She had felt a sense of unreality about it at the time. She made all the arrangements for the abortion herself and was anxious to get it over with and get back to studying for finals. It wasn't until her exams were over that the impact hit her: "I got depressed. I was home for the summer and finally I told my parents. I'm their only daughter and it upset them very much. My mother was sorry I had gone through it without her. She couldn't sleep and cried every time she looked at me, so I ended up consoling her. I'm not telling my parents about the rape. It will hurt them too much. Besides, there is nothing they can do. I may talk to my brother some time, but he lives in California."

The counselor asked if there were other people who were important to her whom she was thinking about telling: "My boyfriend. He's finishing his degree in New York. I've thought about calling him, but I don't want to upset him. I'm going to call him in a couple of days, once I feel ready." The counselor explored Sally's thoughts about how her boyfriend would respond. Sally felt he'd be worried about her and would want to leave school to be with her: "I don't want him to come now. I can handle this myself, and I don't want him to get all upset."

The counselor pointed out that while Sally was worried about others' well-being, including her assailant's, it was very difficult for her to feel comfortable being concerned about herself. Sally agreed. The counselor went on to say that independence was very important to Sally but that she was concerned that Sally felt this meant she couldn't let others help her out. Sally nodded: "I'm the youngest and I guess I feel my parents were very protective of me. My mother especially tried to keep unpleasant things from me. She puts up a front and carries on, while privately she falls apart."

"I wonder if that's not a little like what you are doing?" asked the counselor. Looking a bit surprised, Sally said, "Why, I guess so. I'd get so mad at my mother for doing that—she wouldn't recognize I am an adult and always acted like she had to protect me. Maybe I am doing the same thing."

The counselor suggested that Sally's way of handling her feelings about the rape was to push them aside and to focus on what she could do to protect others. While it was clear that she was very capable, it was as if she wouldn't take the chance of letting anyone see her upset for fear that she would be treated like a little girl again. Sally sighed then and said, "I haven't slept hardly at all for three nights and I'm very nervous about the whole court thing. The DA warned me it could take months, maybe a whole year before it's settled. I don't want to feel this way for a year. I love my job, my life here—I'm scared I'll never feel the same."

This admission led to some specific plans to address her discomfort. Sally was given a prescription for a mild sleeping medication. She said that she had been staying at a different friend's house each night and that she would awaken feeling disoriented. The counselor suggested that she make arrangements to stay in the same place for a few nights. A referral was also made to a witness advocate in the court system who would be available to answer her questions about court and keep her advised about the progress of her case.

As the interview closed, the counselor and Sally agreed to meet for three more times and then to decide if she wished to continue with the counseling. They agreed that the counselor could be useful in helping Sally feel more comfortable acknowledging and attending to her worries about herself. She was given a second appointment in four days and was urged to call should she have any questions or concerns in the meantime.

In the course of the next interview, a second theme emerged. Sally arrived looking more rested and reported that she was sleeping better and thinking of returning home. The counselor reviewed with her the steps she could take to ease her anxiety about being back in her house. These included new locks and having a friend stay with her for a few days. Sally had been considering moving but said, "I love that place and I've been happy there. I'll be damned if I'll let him spoil that for me too." The counselor remarked how angry she sounded.

"I do feel angry, I guess," she said thoughtfully. "It was such a dramatic change in him. I wonder if he can be rehabilitated? I'm worried nothing will be done to help him. He could be acquitted or put on probation since he doesn't have a record. Prison seems useless—it will make him worse. The only thing that will satisfy me is if he's committed to a psychiatric hospital. I think the alcohol triggered the violence in him." The counselor remarked, "At times you sound as if you feel responsible for him."

"I know," Sally said. "Others have said that too. I just believe that people should get help. Who is responsible for him? The defense attorney—he'll try to get him off. His family?" The counselor interjected, "The question is how come *you* feel so responsible?"

Sally replied, "Partly for my safety and the safety of others. I want him taken care of—he needs help. I liked him before. I am angry, but it would be easier if I didn't know him." The counselor asked if this was a dilemma that she had felt in other relationships: Was it difficult for her to get angry? "I don't think so. A few months ago I had a big falling out with a good friend. I felt that the relationship had to end or something had to change, so I confronted her. I could get angry because I was willing to end the relationship. Also, her life would go on fine without me." The counselor observed, "It sounds as if you have to make sure the other person is strong enough before you let yourself get angry."

Sally said, "Maybe. When I get mad about the rape, I can yell or talk to my friends, but I don't have any control over what happens to him. There's no satisfaction in getting mad. I'd just get angrier and more frustrated. I don't want to feel like hitting a wall or killing him." The counselor suggested that many women who are raped have a hard time letting themselves feel angry and that Sally seemed to worry that her anger could hurt the man who raped her. The counselor elaborated, "I wouldn't be surprised if at times you might feel like killing him, but I think the feeling makes you nervous." Sally conceded, "Maybe. But if I got angry where would it go? I don't like feeling angry. He is so pathetic." This led to a discussion about how her protective feelings for him served partly to undo her worry about how angry she could be. They explored how easy it was for her to "nurse" but how anger was antithetical to her image of herself. The counselor suggested that perhaps Sally needed to see her assailant as a sad, pathetic man in order to protect herself from feeling angry and from feeling injured. Sally considered this possibility and related it to some earlier incidents in her family, which confirmed the interpretation.

The rest of the interview and most of the next were spent anticipating her reaction to seeing her assailant again during the probable cause hearing. The theme about being strong, independent, and concerned about others versus feeling injured, needy, and angry was repeatedly discussed. Sally reported that she had made plans to spend the weekend with her boyfriend and was looking forward to getting away. She acknowledged that she was nervous about having sex but had resolved to talk to her boyfriend about it.

Discussion

This summary of the initial phase of the counseling shows the counselor developing a working hypothesis that the rape is stirring up fears about loss of autonomy. These fears are defended against by an intensification of Sally's characterological counterdependent style. Feelings of upset were seen in others to the exclusion of acknowledging her own. Sally had very appropriately taken measures to seek a friend, the police, medical care, and now counseling. She had an available social support system. The risk was that she would push others away in order to fend off the anxiety produced by a revival of her dependency needs. By acknowledging her strengths, the counselor was able to confront Sally with her reluctance to talk about her own needs. The counselor's support of Sally's capabilities and independence made it less threatening for Sally to reveal her anxieties.

The basis of her counterdependency was suggested by the small amount of history elicited. Sally's identification with her mother, her struggle to extricate herself from being the baby in her family, and a persistent underlying conflict about the wish and fear to be protected were assumed to be part of her dynamics. The counselor used this quick assessment to shape her intervention.

Once Sally's concerns about sleep and the court were identified, the counselor attended to them right away. The aim was to help reduce the acute distress and consequently to help Sally fell less needy. This approach also functioned to build an alliance. Contracting to reevaluate the counseling after a limited number of sessions reinforces that the client is in control. In Sally's case, it was an important tactic since she was uncomfortable being on the receiving end of assistance and was worried about being infantilized.

Subsequent interviews demonstrated the development of a solid working alliance, which made it possible for Sally to begin to identify and to work through the feelings stimulated by the rape. Sally's discomfort with her anger was defended against by reaction formation. Her history and associations suggested that guilt about her aggression was a long-standing issue. Sally's inhibition of anger seemed to relate to an unconscious belief that others would be unable to withstand her aggression, and it could presumably be rooted in Sally's experience of her mother as fragile underneath a facade of strength. The counselor made no attempt to pursue this genetic material; instead, she clarified Sally's current uneasiness about being angry at the man who raped her. Thus, the counselor used her understanding of the historical material to make useful clarifications regarding Sally's current difficulties. Sally's reported improvement in sleep and her decision to share with her boyfriend her apprehension about sex are evidence of symptom relief and some modification of her original counterdependent position.

The Working-Through Phase of Counseling

The goals of the working-through phase include increased tolerance of painful affects, symptom relief with restoration of previous functioning, acquisition of new coping skills, and an awareness of how the conscious concerns stimulated by the rape may have roots in earlier basic conflicts. By encouraging a cognitive grasp of how symptoms relate to inner conflicts, the counselor is supporting the victim's self-control (Aguilera & Messick, 1974). Confusion and helplessness will recede. Initially, intervention may be aimed at symptom management. For example, Sally T.'s trepidation about resuming sexual relations with her boyfriend could be approached by first helping her to pinpoint the exact source of her anxiety. For many victims, it is the anticipation of penetration specifically, but the desire remains to be held, cuddled, and kissed. The victim may be encouraged to talk to her partner about what she wants and to explain her discomfort with direct genital contact. Communication with her partner will forestall the development of a pattern of withdrawal from him in order to avoid intercourse. It also reduces the occurrence of unsuccessful attempts, which might reinforce her anxiety and further diminish her self-esteem. If the fear of intercourse persists, the counselor needs to explore for other sources of conflict.

As the middle phase of counseling progresses, repetitive themes will be evident in the victim's material. As this occurs, the counselor may need to adjust her formulation of the initial focus. It is important, however, to relate these themes back to the victim's experience of the rape. Beginning counselors are often dismayed when after the first one or two sessions, the victim stops talking about the rape and shifts to preassault concerns. For example, she may complain about her husband's chronic drinking or reveal that she is having an affair with her married boss.

It is important for the counselor to explore these issues since inevitably they contain elements of the conflict that is stimulated by the rape. The woman upset about her alcoholic husband may be expressing how unavailable he is for her and how unconsciously she blames him for all her troubles, including the rape. The victim having the affair may be harboring guilt about her sexual activity with another woman's husband and may unconsciously experience the rape as punishment for her transgressions. Skillful intervention calls for pointing out how these seemingly extraneous concerns are related to the distress created by the rape. Both of the preceding examples also contain hints of possible underlying psychodynamics. Particularly for counselors used to long-term treatment, there may be a temptation to push toward uncovering these long-standing issues or to make premature and inappropriate interpretations. It is important to respect the boundaries of the counseling contract and to remember that the work is short-term. Historical material and long-standing conflicts should be used to illuminate the rape-related distress (Wolberg, 1965). Long-standing conflicts can be sorted out from the current stress with some awareness of how they are exacerbated by or play into the rape. The counselor can flag them as issues that the victim may choose to work on at some later time.

In the beginning of counseling, when the victim is still raw from the experience of the rape, she is more open to intervention. Her defenses are more fluid, so that both affects and conflicts are more accessible. Roughly four to six weeks after the rape, the acute discomfort usually subsides. Daily functioning gradually returns to normal. There is a retreat from feelings associated with the rape in contrast to the intense preoccupation of the first few weeks. Denial, repression, and rationalization become prominent defenses. Victims talk about how the experience is behind them. Their energy is directed toward the areas of their lives that were temporarily put aside during the initial aftermath of the rape.

This is a time when many victims choose not to continue with counseling. They feel that the need has passed since the subjective discomfort has ended. Some say that they are reluctant to continue for fear the counseling will reawaken now-quiescent concerns. It is important not to struggle with the victim about the need to continue since it will intensify her resistance. It is better to make some predictions about when and how some of her original discomfort may resurface and to keep the door open for her to return. Common precipitants of symptom resurgence are the case's coming to trial, the beginning of a new love relationship, or entry into an unfamiliar situation like starting a new job. It is useful to make an arrangement for a telephone follow-up in a month or so to check on how she is doing.

The time of outward adjustment is greeted by the victim and her family and friends with relief. All concerned wish to erase or undo the tragedy of the rape. The victim's return to normal is tremendously reassuring. Friends and family often support the victim's denial because of their own need to believe that the episode is over and that the effects are gone. If she has taken her case to the police, this is often the time when she wants to drop charges or refuses to testify because she does not want to be reminded of the assault.

The counselor needs to support the victim's accomplishments rather than challenge her position. At the same time, she can clarify the victim's wish to distance herself from the experience and alert her to the likelihood of future concerns. She may caution the victim against making a decision to drop charges immediately and suggest that she wait to see if this decision holds over time. At this juncture, it is also useful to warn family and friends that resolution may not be completed. Victims often feel the loss of attention and sympathy that coincides with symptom relief. No one is around when she wants to talk further about her experience during the process of integration. In fact, others may overtly discourage her from talking and become annoyed when she attempts to do so.

We outline here additional tasks and techniques that become relevant as the counseling process shifts into the working-through phase.

II. *Working-Through Phase of Counseling*
    A. Tasks
        1. *Develop the focus and themes of the victim's concerns.* Establish a working hypothesis about the impact of the rape.
        2. *Identify prior coping measures, both from previous stress situations and from her*

attempts to deal with the rape. Support those skills that have been adaptive and suggest new approaches when indicated.

For example, during her sessions, Barbara D. related that frightening episodes of violence at home had aroused the same helplessness that she had experienced during the rape. She believed that there was nothing she could do to alter the situation with her father, and so she would withdraw and conceal her fear and rage. She explained that she had been very depressed during her adolescence and was feeling even more so after the rape. The counselor suggested that perhaps Barbara's participation in counseling represented an alternate way of coping with her feelings.

3. *Design specific tasks that will increase self-esteem and mastery.* These may include introspection and reflection, such as "When you wake up in the middle of the night, I'd like you to pay attention to what you are thinking or try to recall if you had a dream so that we can talk about it next time." Obviously, tasks can be specific actions that need to be taken. For example, one may encourage the victim to arrange for the landlord to install new locks, to make a transcript of the rape incident for further court appearances, or to approach her professor to arrange an extension on a paper.

4. *Support the use of family and friends as resources.* The victim's anxiety usually decreases once she has been able to talk with the people who matter to her the most. Reality-test the feelings of mistrust or criticism she may be experiencing from others. Reiterate willingness to meet with them.

B. Techniques

1. *Openly express encouragement and interest.*

2. *Use anticipatory guidance.* Help prepare the victim for what she can do to handle situations that are likely to provoke anxiety, such as court appearances or being alone in her apartment.

Barbara D. felt much trepidation about men in general and wondered whether she could ever date a man comfortably. Toward the end of her therapy, she was asked out and decided to go. Before this date, Barbara was filled with fantasies that this man would assault her. The counselor helped her to reality-test these fantasies and to consider what she could do to control her anxiety. Barbara decided that she would feel safest in a public place with her date and suggested that they go to the movies. She later told the counselor that enjoying the date was enormously reassuring to her.

3. *Gently confront resistances when they appear.* For example, when the victim comes late to an appointment following a session in which she got angry for the first time, suggest that she may have been made anxious by those feelings and so comes late to avoid experiencing them again.

4. *Explicitly deal with transference when it threatens to impede progress.* It is not uncommon for a victim to project superego censure onto the counselor. She might think that the counselor blames her for the rape, just as she experienced her mother as critical and disapproving whenever she went to her with a problem. Obviously, the counselor needs to be clear that her own countertransference is not being acted out and that indeed it is a projection, before she interprets this to the victim.

5. *Adjust activity to the needs of the victim.* As the victim becomes mobilized, the counselor shifts to a less directive approach and reinforces the victim's increasing sense of autonomy.

Case Example: Sally T.

Sally opened the fourth interview by saying that the weekend with her boyfriend had gone well. She felt relieved in talking to him and by the end of the visit had felt comfortable having sex, which was reassuring to both of them. She quickly went on to talk about her reaction to seeing her assailant during the probable cause hearing. She reported that he did not look sad and pathetic as she had imagined but rather appeared to be without remorse. "Once I saw that, I changed from feeling 90% sad to feeling 90% angry," Sally stated. She went on to describe the questions asked by the defense attorney that were aimed at developing a defense of consent: "He asked me if I enjoyed it; he asked how he got my legs apart. I was furious. But the anger got me through it—it gave me strength. Damn it, I wasn't going to let him make a fool of me."

Both the district attorney and the police detective had commented that they thought her assailant's attorney wasn't very competent: "They said it to reassure me about a conviction, but it got me worried. I still feel he needs help. I'm going to give my recommendation to the trial judge. Overall, though, I feel better. Some definite action is being taken. It's also freeing to feel angry instead of responsible." Her counselor acknowledged how difficult it was to testify and how well she had handled it. She then underscored the strength Sally experienced from feeling her anger. "Perhaps your sense of responsibility about him was weighted by having to keep your anger hidden," the counselor suggested.

Sally went on to discuss how her friends at work didn't appreciate how upset she was because she was functioning well. She remarked, "I'm learning a lot about how I cope. I don't let many people see how I really feel. I've been trying to be more straightforward with my friends because I don't want to go though this alone."

Toward the end of the session, her thoughts returned to her assailant: "Ever since the hearing I've been feeling scared that he will come and hurt me. I imagine he hates me for telling on him." The counselor reviewed how when she was feeling sad and sorry for him, she imagined him to be pathetic and remorseful. Now that she was angry, she imagined him to be angry, too. Sally replied, "When I felt he was sad, I felt safe. But now I've done something—I've testified against him." The counselor pointed out that her worry about retaliation seemed to come from her discomfort about her own aggression. "Yes, but when I get angry I don't get violent; he does!" Sally exclaimed. The counselor agreed but wondered if there was still some guilt she felt about being angry. The counselor went over the fact that the assailant had known since his arrest that she was taking action and that the turning point in feeling unsafe coincided with Sally's beginning to feel angry. She considered this possibility and agreed. This exchange led to a discussion about whether Sally wished to continue with counseling. Her uneasiness about being angry, her continuing anxiety about being alone, and her worries about the court were identified as areas that she wished to work on in the process of reviewing her progress to date.

The next two sessions centered on feelings of vulnerability precipitated by an obscene phone call. She initially worried that it was connected with the rape but eventually concluded that it was coincidental. Sally described feeling a sense of loss because she was no longer carefree and confident. She cataloged the precautions she now took. In addition to encouraging her to report the call to the police and to change her phone number, the counselor supported the adaptive side of her increased vigilance. She also reassured Sally that the intensity of her anxiety would gradually diminish. Sally's feeling of vulnerability brought up how in the past, she had hidden such feelings from others because of her uneasiness in being "smothered" with concern. She gradually became more at ease with taking support from her friends. The way in which this vulnerability was also connected with her anticipation of punishment for feeling angry and taking court action against the assailant was repeatedly discussed.

During the seventh session, Sally reported that a trial date had been set three months hence. She was both relieved to have a definite end point in sight and nervous about the trial itself. She said that she was feeling much better, was less anxious about being alone, and was feeling much less worried about retaliation: "You know, the more I talk about how unfair it was to have my whole life turned around by the rape and the more I can get mad at that guy, the less depressed I feel." Sally said that while she wished to continue counseling until the trial, she didn't feel that she needed to come every week. She and the counselor worked out a plan to meet in two weeks and then once a month until the trial. The counselor made it clear that Sally could call any time she felt the need.

The three subsequent visits focused on clarifying and elaborating the issues laid out in prior sessions. Sally reported a steady decline in her preoccupation about the rape. "I mainly think about it when I come to see you," she said. "I've got my energy back and am up to my ears with my work." Sally also reported that she and her boyfriend were talking about living together once he finished his degree in the spring. She was very excited about that and pleased with her capacity to get on with her life.

As the trial date drew closer, there was a recurrence of some symptoms: sleep loss, increased startle reactions, suspiciousness of strange men, and fear of retaliation by the assailant. The counselor urged Sally to think about what was most worrisome about the trial. At the same time, she reassured Sally that the symptom return was not unusual. The connection between feeling vulnerable and her guilt about being angry and taking aggressive action by testifying again emerged. In the meantime, Sally had met with a witness advocate and her DA to go over her testimony for the trial.

Sally called after the trial date to make an appointment. She said that she thought this would be her last session. She arrived announcing how relieved she felt. Her assailant had pleaded guilty and received a 10-year sentence. She acknowledged that she had mixed feelings about the outcome. She remarked, "You know, it's funny, I think I still have some guilt about his needing psychiatric help and fear about his seeking revenge, but it doesn't feel the same. I really feel it was worth sticking through this. You really have to be strong to do it."

The counselor reinforced this conclusion and asked about whether there had been any change in her symptoms. Sally reported that she was sleeping fine now but still got anxious when she saw someone who physically resembled her assailant: "But I feel as if it's under control. The crazy thing is that since the trial is over, I'm more emotional about the rape. Like I'll cry more easily, which I didn't do before. It's as if now I can allow myself to really feel it, whereas before I felt I had to be in control for court."

The counselor replied that being in control didn't have to mean denying her feelings. She added, "It takes time to put this experience in perspective, and you will probably continue to feel sad and angry and some of the guilt for a while." They reviewed what Sally had accomplished over the course of the counseling. Sally said, "I feel kind of sad saying good-bye to you. But I really do feel I can manage fine now. The irony is that I feel stronger having weathered this experience. The biggest change is that it's much easier for me to let my friends in on how I'm feeling without getting so nervous about it." The counselor remarked, "I guess you've learned that being strong doesn't mean you can't ask for a helping hand along the way. It takes a special kind of strength to give others the chance to be supportive, especially when you're used to being the one giving out the help." Sally nodded; then she laughed: "You know, I've even been considering telling my parents some day. I'm not sure I will, but I don't feel so strongly that it would be a disaster. I have handled this well and I know that. Now I believe my parents would see that too." The session ended with good-byes.

Discussion

The main task of the working-through phase was to increase Sally's ability to tolerate feeling angry and vulnerable. The counselor was active in clarifying how her fear of retaliation escalated once she began to feel angry at her assailant. Sally projected her hostility onto the man and then was frightened that he would become violent toward her. When she felt sad, she believed he was sad, and she felt safe. The counselor understood that Sally's feeling responsible for the assailant was partially determined by her guilt about her own aggression. However, there was no attempt to uncover how this dynamic operated in other relationships or to explore its etiology in the past.

The obscene phone call intensified Sally's worry that the world was dangerous. The counselor was again active in identifying and supporting the steps that Sally might take to protect herself. The phone call and the probable cause hearing were both stressful events that recapitulated elements of the original assault. They provided the opportunity to rework the experience of being intruded on, fearful and helpless, one step removed from the rape itself.

Sally's use of friends as a source of comfort became less conflicted as her self-esteem stabilized. By consistently treating her as a responsible adult, the counselor diminished her concerns about being treated as a child. Fortunately, Sally's friends were responsive and her experience with the police and district attorney was positive, so that her openness was reinforced. When this is not the case, the counselor may need to intervene directly with the social system.

The frequency of the counseling sessions was geared to the need of the client. As Sally felt growing confidence in her capacity to manage, the counselor adjusted her activity to allow Sally to exercise her autonomy. The resurgence of symptoms around the trial was handled as an expectable and temporary regression. Because of the pride she derived from her successful management of the stresses following the rape, Sally's self-esteem was enhanced. Although she continued to have some anxiety, her defenses were more flexible, and her appraisal of herself and others had become more realistic. When she and her counselor parted, both felt sure of Sally's capacity to resolve her feelings about the rape and to integrate the assault as a tragic but accepted part of her life.

The Termination Phase of Counseling

The final stage of counseling is geared to making explicit which coping measures have been useful for the victim. While the immediate gains of short-term work are usually modest, hopefully the victim will have acquired the skills and confidence to continue on her own to resolve her feelings about the rape. It is our impression that rape work, like grief work, takes approximately two years to complete. An intrinsic part of that process involves the victim's mourning the loss of her former image of herself and her social environment. It is not unusual for a victim to express the feeling that she has lost her childhood innocence. She can no longer pretend that she is inviolable; her human frailty is poignantly clear. Fellow human beings can no longer be regarded as unquestionably benign or trustworthy. The rape and its effects on the victim's self-image, relationships, and expectations of the world take time to be accepted and integrated. The counselor offers support, direction, and a relationship in which to begin the process.

The working-through phase of the counseling facilitates symptom relief and restores the victim to her previous level of functioning. Optimally, the victim will have increased her capacity to tolerate confusing and painful affects and will have expanded her repertoire of coping mechanisms. She will have a greater understanding of her characterological conflicts and how they were activated by the trauma. In the final stage of the counseling, the victim reevaluates her responses to the assault and her progress during the course of treatment. She prepares to terminate her work with the counselor and anticipates how she will manage with future stress.

The termination phase is usually accompanied by a regression that recapitulates some of the concerns, symptoms, and behavior that the victim originally presented. Powerful feelings may resurface as she again confronts the question she posed in her initial anguish: "Why did this have to happen to me?" This temporary regression provides the victim with an opportunity to reexperience the assault one step removed, and in the reassuring presence of her counselor. With the counselor's support and clarification, and using the new perspective and skills she has acquired, the victim attempts to master the experience once more before she is on her own. If the counseling has been successful, she will have come to feel proud of her demonstrated ability to survive and master a major life stress.

During the termination, the victim must also face losing the counselor with whom she has shared her personal tragedy. Giving up the counselor is particularly difficult for those victims who lack support outside the counseling relationship. In contrast to Sally T., Barbara D.'s family relationships were too disturbed for her to utilize in a growth-promoting way. The rape had temporarily confirmed her belief that men are irrational and violent and women passive and masochistic. Reaching out to her parents felt like a regressive step to her, but at the time of termination, she had no other friends to support her attempt to view relationships in a new way. It was with considerable pain that Barbara D. terminated her therapy, and she used her last sessions to discuss feeling angry and depressed because she could never rely on her parents.

For most victims, memories of previous losses are stimulated along with earlier conflicts about dependency needs. Sometimes victims become anxious that they will lose the gains they have made when the counselor is no longer available. As the ending date approaches, the victim may begin emphasizing what a difficult time she is still having, or she may introduce a new array of concerns. It is important that the counselor point out the victim's reluctance to stop treatment and address her concerns in the context of the loss of the counseling relationship. This is also the time when the counselor needs to underscore what activities, insights, and approaches the victim has undertaken on her own behalf. Long-standing problems should again be labeled, and the victim should be reminded that she may choose to seek psychotherapy in the future.

Sometimes, the victim is not alone in her difficulty saying good-bye. The counselor may discover that it is hard to let her go because of the bond forged in sharing the crisis. Rape victims are often very gratifying clients to work with because they get better. The counselor may be tempted to open up other areas for examination or "forget" to remind the victim of their termination date. She may find herself becoming apprehensive about the victim's being on her own, or she may lose her perspective on the nature and function of the victim's regression during this phase. It is very important that the counselor be aware of the possibility of these reactions and not act them out by prolonging the relationship. In most instances, such a prolongation serves only to confirm the victim's doubts about her capacity to manage effectively on her own. In some instances, however, it may be appropriate to continue the treatment. It is the counselor's responsibility to make a sound clinical assessment separate from the resistance she or the victim may feel about termination. While Barbara D. presented many other long-standing difficulties, including a highly ambivalent relationship with her parents, poor object choices, and a characterological depression, she and the counselor decided to stick to their original short-term contract. They agreed that at the time of termination, Barbara's confidence in her ability to function autonomously took precedence over these other issues. Barbara decided to attend school for another year and then to review her need for further treatment.

As with the termination of any psychotherapy, the counselor must be prepared to deal with transference and other resistances. For example, a victim may experience the ending of the counseling as a desertion. Angry feelings about the depriving counselor or self-castigation about not having been a "good" client can emerge as the affective explanation for the termination. The victim may begin to come late to the interviews or forget appointments. These reactions must be dealt with directly, and once again, the counselor should aim to reinforce the victim's sense of competency.

During the termination, it is important for the victim to make a realistic appraisal of the limitations of both the counseling and the counselor. This appraisal often involves making explicit her unspoken wishes that the counselor would protect and take care of her or that the counseling could magically erase the rape from her life. She will experience some disappointment about what was not accomplished in counseling as well as feelings of gratitude toward the counselor and relief that the trauma is behind her. A review of the victim's progress should include areas of continuing concern as well as her accomplishments. Future difficulties need to be anticipated, and the counselor should warn the victim to expect some setbacks. The task is to encourage future planning that applies the understanding and coping strategies the victim has learned during the counseling process.

Rape counseling challenges the clinician's ability to deal with powerful affects, to make skilled diagnostic assessments and therapeutic interventions, and to engage the victim in a trusting relationship. The positive impact of making a meaningful contact with the victim cannot be underestimated. An encounter in which the counselor demonstrates respect and empathy for the victim is often the first step toward helping her to restore a positive sense of self-worth and faith in mutual caring relationships. Within the context of this kind of supportive relationship, the victim can be mobilized to actively master the trauma and its sequelae. In fact, the rape crisis can act as a catalyst for further growth that is supported by, but does not end with, the counseling process. It is a testimony to human endurance and energy that even the most painful of tragedies can be transformed into a positive turning point in one's life.

References

Aguilera, D., & Messick, J. *Crisis intervention theory and methodology.* St. Louis: C. V. Mosby Company, 1974.

Brownmiller, S. *Against our will: Men, women and rape.* New York: Simon & Schuster, 1975.

Burgess, A. W., & Holmstrom, L. L. Rape trauma syndrome. *American Journal of Psychiatry,* September 1974, *131,* 981–986. (a)

Burgess, A. W., & Holmstrom, L. L. *Rape: Victims of crisis.* Bowie, Md.: Robert J. Brady Company, 1974. (b)

Golan, N. When is a client in crisis? *Social Casework,* July 1969, *50*(7), 389–394.

Golan, N. *Treatment in crisis situations.* New York: The Free Press, 1978.

Haley, S. When the patient reports atrocities. *Archives of General Psychiatry,* February 1974, *30,* 191–196.

Horowitz, M. *Stress response syndromes.* New York: Jason Aronson Inc., 1976.

Lindemann, E. Symptomatology and management of acute grief. *American Journal of Psychiatry,* 1944, *101,* 141–148.

McCombie, S. Characteristics of rape victims seen in crisis intervention. *Smith College Studies in Social Work,* March 1976, *46,* 137–158.

Smith, L. A review of crisis intervention theory. *Social Casework,* July 1978, 396–405.

Sutherland, S., & Scherl, D. Patterns of response among victims of rape. *American Journal of Orthopsychiatry,* April 1970, *40*(3), 503–511.

Titchener, J., & Kapp, F. Family and character change at Buffalo Creek. *American Journal of Psychiatry,* March 1976, *133*(3), 764–769.

Wolberg, L. R. (Ed.). *Short-term psychotherapy.* New York: Grune & Stratton, 1965.

Zonderman, S. A study of volunteer rape crisis counselors. Master's thesis, Smith College School of Social Work, 1975.

12

Counseling the Mates and Families of Rape Victims

DANIEL SILVERMAN AND SHARON L. MCCOMBIE

Male mates and family members may find it difficult to respond to the female rape victim in an empathic and supportive manner for a variety of cognitive and emotional reasons. The purpose of this chapter is to describe common patterns of reaction among the husbands, boyfriends, and family members of rape victims; to outline the dynamics of such responses and their effects on the relationships involved; and to offer technical suggestions to the counselor, who must deal not only with the intense feelings of mates and family members but also with his or her own emotional responses to the affectively laden topic of rape victimization.

Increasing clinical experience in rape crisis counseling has led to the inescapable conclusion that therapeutic and didactic work with mates and family members may be critical in attempts to help the victim (Silverman, 1977). Just as rape represents a traumatic event that precipitates a crisis in the life of the victim, it may also assault the psychological equilibrium of the victim's couple and family systems. Abrupt changes in the balance of interpersonal relations and family functions may occur in direct parallel to the intrapsychic disharmony experienced by the rape victim. There are four important ways in which counseling interventions may be indispensable in

DANIEL SILVERMAN, M.D. ● Instructor in Psychiatry, Harvard Medical School; Director of Medical Education, Department of Psychiatry, Beth Israel Hospital, Boston, Massachusetts. SHARON L. MCCOMBIE, M.S.W., A.C.S.W. ● Founder and Director, Rape Crisis Intervention Program, Beth Israel Hospital; Clinical Instructor, Simmons College School of Social Work, Boston, Massachusetts.

This chapter has been adapted, with permission, from "Sharing the Crisis of Rape: Counseling the Mates and Families of Victims," *American Journal of Orthopsychiatry*, 1978, 48(1), 166–173. Copyright 1978, The American Orthopsychiatric Association, Inc.

assisting mates and family members to provide a truly supportive environment for the victim's reconstitutive efforts in the posttraumatic period: (1) by encouraging the open expression on the part of mates and family members of their affective responses to this shared life crisis; (2) by facilitating cognitive understanding of what the experience of rape actually represents to the victim; (3) by educating the people close to the victim about the nature of the crisis she's experiencing and helping them to anticipate future likely psychological and somatic sequelae of the traumatic episode (Burgess & Holmstrom, 1974a); and (4) by providing direct counseling services to individual family members whose personal responses to the shared crisis are so profound as to affect their ability to cope adaptively.

Persons close to the female rape victim may be subject to the same misunderstandings, prejudices, and mythologies surrounding the crime of rape held by the general public (Amir, 1971). A common tendency in this regard is that of reacting more to the sexual than to the inherently violent aspects of the rape. To understand the responses of male mates or family members, it is important to remember that they may be firmly of the opinion that "Nice women don't get raped," "Only sexy young women are ever raped," or "Any woman who is raped must have asked for it" (Bassuk, Savitz, McCombie, & Pell, 1975). Such thoughts are inevitably linked with feelings of resentment and anger toward the victim, although the individual may not be consciously aware of it. One boyfriend of a rape victim, when asked if he believed his girlfriend to be in any way responsible for her rape revealed his unconscious feelings when he remarked emphatically, "Of course not! I have no doubt she *was* responsible." Not surprisingly, feelings of anger toward the victim are expressed openly only with considerable difficulty and often are manifested indirectly. Subtle derivatives of angry feelings may be observed in doubting the veracity of the victim's story; criticizing the woman for "not having been more careful," even when it's clear that carelessness played no part in precipitating the rape; or wondering whether she "enjoyed" the experience. One husband was distraught to learn that his wife had experienced an orgasm during the rape and felt enraged because he was certain that he "would never be able to give her as exciting a sexual experience again." It is possible that this man's anger served to defend against the emergence of difficult feelings about his own sexual adequacy and an unfavorable comparison with the rapist, who was viewed as possessing special prowess.

While the basis of such feelings may be understandable, the critical problem here is, very simply, that such attitudes and the emotions they generate make the "revictimization" of the woman a real possibility. Counselors must be alert to the presence of such misapprehensions and their associated feelings and work gently to mobilize them into direct expression. This is crucial, as the unearthing of such feelings and their causes allows for far greater control of the potentially damaging covert or mixed communications that they may engender between the victim and her male mate. Individual sessions with husband or boyfriend may allow the emergence and clarification of such material in an environment of safety, privacy, and confidentiality for the man and protection for the absent victim.

Another attitude commonly expressed by boyfriends and husbands is the view of the woman as the "property of her man" (Brownmiller, 1975). Male mates may feel personally wronged and attacked by the rape of "their woman" and may display a proprietary indignation that serves more to protect against their own unconscious sense of vulnerability than to express a deeply held personal philosophy. It is important for the counselor to realize that these feelings are multiply determined. They may reflect common male attitudes about feminine sexuality, the veneration of virginity, and a sense of entitlement to "exclusive rights" to that sexuality. More deeply, however, there may be unconscious concerns about homosexuality stirred by having been "had" by the rapist when "he took my woman" or discomfort associated with the excitement of "sharing a woman with another man." Other misapprehensions that may impede supportive behavior on the part of male mates include anger over the fact that the victim has "allowed herself" to become "devalued" or "damaged merchandise" (Sutherland & Scherl, 1970). One boyfriend wondered whether he would ever be able to escape the thought that his girlfriend was "tainted" by her experience. Another felt that his lover would bear a permanent stigma, "like a scarlet R on her forehead." A husband described feeling physically disgusted when approaching his "unclean" wife sexually, immediately following her rape. Obviously, such responses may reinforce the victim's sense of humiliation and devaluation.

A potential difficulty for the counselor is the negative personal reactions such "unenlightened" or "chauvinistic" feelings may evoke. Being openly critical of the man for having these feelings is only likely to heighten his sense of feeling attacked, which may already be present as a result of identification with the loved one. It may serve to further increase defensiveness and anger, and decrease the opportunity for the useful ventilation of the affects. A helpful counseling maneuver could be to focus supportively on the man's injury as a result of the rape of his mate, suggesting that whenever a loved one suffers a trauma or loss of any kind (e.g., through illness or injury), he too experiences pain and loss. Furthermore, mates and family members should be helped to realize that while rape is a terribly traumatic experience with sequelae not unlike a grief reaction (Lindemann, 1944), the victim need not be permanently debilitated by it. It may be useful to explain that while an individual may never "forget" unfortunate or tragic experiences such as the death of a beloved person, these memories do not make it impossible to go on living a rich and satisfying life after an adequate opportunity to mourn the loss.

Perhaps the most important point to be made here is that the counselor must remember that the mate's frustrations may grow out of a shared sense of devaluation and shame. One woman's husband, depressed and tearful, expressed this clearly when he remarked, "I feel as if I'd been raped too." Mates must be allowed to discuss difficult feelings fully in an atmosphere of noncritical acceptance and understanding. Only then should the counselor consider beginning didactic work to disabuse the man of his misconceptions.

The importance of involving the male partner of the rape victim in cases of stable or married couples cannot be stressed enough. The crisis precipitated by rape is a mutual one, and the man is potentially his mate's prime support. Clearly, the rape experience stresses vulnerable areas in any relationship (Notman & Nadelson, 1976). For example, the sense that the man failed to protect his woman from being raped could precipitate feelings in the victim or the mate about how good a protector or provider the man is in general. Couples whose sexual relations have been problematic prior to the rape are likely to experience considerable new stress in that area, and this aspect of the relationship may have to be carefully explored and evaluated by the counselor to determine whether specific therapeutic intervention for sexual dysfunction is needed. In some cases, the rape may serve as a catalyst that crystallizes previously unaddressed conflicts. In others, it may stimulate a total reevaluation of the quality of the relationship and precipitate a newfound closeness and common sense of purpose in response to the external crisis the couple shares. The goal of counseling interventions for couples, then, is to make these facts conscious and explicit so that the closeness may be solidified and adaptive strategies brought under voluntary control. In situations where the rape experience unearths significant individual or couples' issues of long standing, it may be necessary to allow the crisis intervention to develop into a more traditional ongoing counseling experience or to refer the victim or couple for longer-term therapy. Clearly, such clinical decisions must be made on a case-by-case basis in harmony with the needs, wishes, and motivations of the clients.

In the acute posttraumatic period, parents and siblings of rape victims may experience a sense of shock, helplessness, rage, or physical revulsion that parallels the affective responses of the victim (Sutherland & Scherl, 1970). Immediately following her rape, one father drove his daughter over to the apartment of a friend who had also been a rape victim because "she seemed so helpless; I felt so helpless. I didn't know what to say, and the only thing I could think of to do was to get her to talk to her friend."

In their anxiety to help the victim and contain their own feelings of helplessness, families may attempt to rally the support of the victim's women and men friends, clergy, co-workers, teachers, supervisors, and so on. At times, particularly in the acute posttraumatic period, the woman may experience these attempts as invasive. The woman may still be in a period of relative denial of what has happened to her or may wish to share the reality with only a chosen few. Her need for privacy and confidentiality or simply her reticence to discuss her crisis at all must be respected by families and helping professionals alike. The family may find it useful to ventilate their concerns and sense of frustration over being unable to help "undo" the victim's plight by talking to the counselor in the victim's absence. This may be particularly important in those situations where victims refuse any follow-up contact with rape counseling services because of their need to deny difficult feelings of vulnerability and helplessness. Families may use counseling services in these situations to understand the basis of the woman's resistance to counseling as well as to develop useful strategies for assisting the victim in absentia through their supportive efforts.

Fathers, brothers, and mates of victims may experience frequent thoughts of extracting violent retribution from the rapist on behalf of the woman. One brother of a rape victim spoke in lurid detail of how he would "rip the s.o.b. apart with my bare hands" if given the opportunity. These thoughts may function to protect the man against his own sense of utter helplessness and the impotent rage he shares, albeit unconsciously, with the victim. In some cases, the underlying dynamic of powerful fantasies of revenge may be an attempt to "act out" the woman's desire to see her victimizer suffer in the way she has. Ironically, this may result in the woman's having to bear the additional burden of calming, placating, and reassuring the men who would be her avenging protectors. Counselors should be alert to this situation and ready to point out the potential disservice done the victim by the man's overzealousness.

The above reactions on the part of family members seem to represent an affective identification with the victim, as well as personal responses and attempts to cope with the stress of the life crisis they are sharing with the victim. In some cases of rape, interpersonal difficulties in the form of intense parent–child or couples' conflicts seem to lead individuals to place themselves at greater risk of personal harm. People who care less about themselves because of disordered relationships tend to take less care of themselves. One woman, angry at her husband because of his late working hours and unavailability, left their apartment following a heated argument, insisting on taking the dog out alone at 2:00 A.M. During this unprecedented late-night walk, she was raped in the unlit public park in which she sat. A 17-year-old woman, following an especially vitriolic exchange with her parents over independence and life-style, stormed from her home in the late evening and, for the first time, hitchhiked alone to a dance that her parents had demanded she forgo. She was raped by the young occupants of the car who had picked her up. In both cases, the family members of the rape victim experienced considerable guilt and sense of responsibility for precipitating the rape. Anger with the victim for "retaliating by getting herself hurt" was clearly present as well. (In difficult situations like this, the counselor must help sort out responsibility and clarify the way in which the conflicts and events leading up to the rape may have reflected self-destructive attempts to deal with ongoing interpersonal problems.)

Families often mobilize themselves to cope with the crisis precipitated by rape in predictable ways. Patronization and overprotection in the aftermath of a rape are common responses. Immediately following her rape, one woman's parents quickly rented an apartment in "a good neighborhood where they couldn't afford to send me before" and moved her belongings there. Another family of a woman who had been assaulted in her own apartment insisted on chauffeuring their daughter by car to and from work, to the store, and to visit friends despite the fact that she had previously lived alone and used public transportation. Other families urge victims to move to a new city or to return home, "where we can watch you and keep you safe." These maneuvers may represent an attempt on the part of the family members to assuage feelings of guilt and responsibility for having failed to protect the "defenseless" woman from being raped in the first place. While such gestures of concern are undoubtedly well-intentioned, there is a ready danger in such actions because they may communicate the idea to the victim that important people in her life see her as a vulnerable child in need of caretaking. This view can reinforce the victim's own sense of "I am indeed helpless and defenseless" and prevent her from using her more adaptive strategies for coping with the crisis, strategies that might not be as regressive or costly in terms of self-esteem and sense of autonomy. Counseling interventions that support the family's earnest desire to be caretaking and helpful but that also indicate the counterproductiveness of infantilizing the victim are important contributions.

Another coping tactic used by families is distraction. The idea here is to keep the victim occupied with group activities, vacation trips, shopping sprees, and the like in an attempt to deny and undo the effects of the rape. In some situations, in direct contrast to overinvolvement and intrusiveness, the victim may be encouraged by her mate or one member of the family to keep the rape a "secret between us" to "protect" other family members from being traumatized. Examples of this include "protecting Mother from upset," "not letting Dad know because he will be enraged" with the victim, or "sheltering" younger siblings or children if the victim is a mother. As is generally the case, family "secrets" tend to become great burdens and can be destructive of potentially adaptive behaviors. The reasons for a conspiracy of silence vary, but they may include parental discomfort with one's own or the child's sexuality, fear of blame for negligence, or simply hidden alliances and long-standing family problems. Obviously, chronically disturbed family relationships may impede supportive efforts as much as the foregoing specific maladaptive family responses to the rape crisis. Attempts either to hide the truth or to distract one from it, are based on the family's conviction that open, ongoing discussion of the trauma keeps painful, disorganizing memories alive in a destructive way. The impact of such a stance is to deprive the woman of the opportunity to mourn the personal loss inherent in her rape experience, to deny her much-needed support, and to communicate by inference that "What's happened is simply too terrible to discuss," confirming the victim's worst fears and doubts.

As indicated earlier, a significant component of the counseling intervention with families and mates of rape victims must be educational. Following an opportunity to discuss fully the difficult kinds of feelings described above in an atmosphere of noncritical acceptance, the counselor should make efforts to teach the family and the mate about the nature of the crisis precipitated by rape. The focus should be on the following four points.

1. The counselor should explain the inherently violent nature of rape as a crime, helping family members to understand that the victim's experience has been more of a threat to life than a sexual episode. It must be made clear that the predominant feelings experienced by victims posttraumatically are powerlessness in the face of a life-and-death situation, vulnerability, devaluation, and fear of loss of ability to control the events in their lives (Sutherland & Scherl, 1970). Family members may need considerable assistance in helping the victim to remobilize her most effective coping behaviors. Understanding the kinds of feelings she is experiencing is a crucial first step in laying the groundwork for family responses that will not undermine the woman's attempts to help herself. In addition, families may require guidance in identifying and demythologizing long-held attitudes about women who are raped. Using one's position as an authoritative but nonpunitive teacher with a fund of knowledge concerning the crime of rape (Burgess & Holmstrom, 1974a,b; Amir, 1971; Brownmiller, 1975; Sutherland & Scherl, 1970; Schultz, 1975), the counselor can do much to disabuse families and mates of their misunderstanding and biases.

2. The counselor should prepare the family for the predictable psychological and physiological sequelae of the rape, described as the *rape trauma syndrome* (Burgess & Holmstrom, 1974a). He or she should explain carefully in advance that following a period of apparent outward readjustment, there may be an emergence of nightmares, insomnia, somatic symptoms, anxiety attacks, phobias, depression, crying, and, more significantly, feelings of fear, humiliation, anger, and self-blame. Foreknowledge of these possible reaction patterns may help to lessen family members' concern when they occur and allow them to respond to the victim in a more calm and reassuring manner.

3. The counselor should help the family understand that they are most productive when they assist the woman in mobilizing her own best coping

abilities (Burgess & Holmstrom, 1976) as an autonomous adult rather than treating her as a sheltered child. This approach includes encouraging the family to allow, but not force, the open expression of the victim's feelings; conveying strongly the idea that rape, like other life crises, need not destroy the woman's potential for normal functioning in the future; and helping the family learn how to control their desires to intervene forcefully to "undo" the rape trauma.

4. Most importantly, the counselor should teach the family and mate the concept of "containment" of the victim's feelings. This means explaining how to provide an accepting and safe "holding environment" (Winnicott, 1965) into which the woman can release her troubling thoughts and feelings without fear of condemnation or critical response born of a shared sense of helplessness. The counselor, by way of example, must model containing behaviors of empathy, willingness to address difficult material with poise, gentle reassurance, and an avoidance of the tendency to be overly directive. This approach implies helping the family to grasp the very difficult reality that there is no single magical or right thing that can be said or done to make "everything better." The counselor must not only share the family's disappointment over this unfortunate fact but also help them to realize that in being emotionally available to, caring of, and genuinely concerned about the woman, they are offering her much that is immediately invaluable and eventually restorative.

The crucial point to be made is the absolute necessity of involving important members of the victim's social network in the postrape counseling intervention. The mobilization of decisive support and help with guided family participation is critical, and the potential for increased burdening and revictimization of the woman is considerable if such efforts are lacking.

Interventions follow two distinct tacks: (1) facilitating the expression of emotional response to the shared life crisis and (2) disabusing misconception and preparing for constructive strategies of coping through education about the nature of the crisis. Typical crisis responses of mates and family members are observable, and foreknowledge of these patterns may be extremely helpful to the counselor in determining and individualizing clinical approaches and maneuvers. A summary of the kinds of responses seen can be made following Lazarus's behavioral classification of coping reaction patterns (1966), which includes (1) actions aimed at strengthening the individual's resources against harm, (2) avoidance, (3) attack, and (4) inaction. Examples of the first category include seeking out and obtaining postrape counseling and gynecological services, joining rape victim support groups, family attempts to protect the woman, physical relocation, or the highly adaptive behavior of cooperation with the criminal justice system to ultimately remove rapists from the general population. Avoidance is seen in the techniques of distraction or the maintenance of a conspiracy of silence.

Attacking behavior may be represented in the stimulation of fantasies of retribution, blaming the victim, or the displacement of anger onto would-be helpers exhibited by some victims. Inaction, in the form of failure to avail oneself of professional counseling and medical assistance, is both potentially dangerous and tragic in its consequences.

The most significant idea that the counselor can share with his or her clients is containment of the difficult human emotions provoked by rape victimization. To a great extent, this is done more by deed than word and demands that the counselor attain a considerable knowledge of and be comfortable in dealing with the affectively charged crisis of rape.

References

Amir, M. *Patterns of forcible rape.* Chicago: University of Chicago Press, 1971.

Bassuk, E., Savitz, R., McCombie, S., & Pell, S. Organizing a rape crisis program in a general hospital. *Journal of the American Medical Women's Association,* 1975, *30,* 486–490.

Brownmiller, S. *Against our will: Men, women and rape.* New York: Simon & Schuster, 1975.

Burgess, A. W., & Holmstrom, L. L. Rape trauma syndrome. *American Journal of Psychiatry,* 1974, *131,* 981–986. (a)

Burgess, A. W., & Holmstrom, L. L. *Rape: Victims of crisis.* Bowie, Md.: Robert J. Brady Company, 1974. (b)

Burgess, A. W., & Holmstrom, L. L. Coping behavior of the rape victim. *American Journal of Psychiatry,* 1976, *133,* 413–418.

Lazarus, R. S. *Psychological stress and the coping process.* New York: McGraw-Hill Book Company, 1966.

Lindemann, E., Symptomatology and management of acute grief. *American Journal of Psychiatry,* 1944, *101,* 141–156.

Notman, M., & Nadelson, C. The rape victim: Psychodynamic considerations. *American Journal of Psychiatry,* 1976, *133,* 408–412.

Schultz, L. G. (Ed.). *Rape victimology.* Springfield, Ill., Charles C Thomas, 1975.

Silverman, D. First do no more harm: Female rape victims and the male counselor. *American Journal of Orthopsychiatry,* 1977, *47,* 91–96.

Sutherland, S., & Scherl, D. Patterns of response among victims of rape. *American Journal of Orthopsychiatry,* 1970, *40,* 503–511.

Winnicott, D. W. *The maturational process and the facilitating environment.* New York: International Universities Press, 1965.

VI

Special Considerations

This last section deals with two separate subjects that could not be easily classified within the other sections of the handbook. They are, however, important aspects of rape crisis intervention. The treatment of the child victim is a complicated subject that deserves a separate volume. We have included an introductory discussion to familiarize the reader with some of the main issues that vary from the treatment of the adult victim. The Silverman chapter covers the frequently neglected area of the male counselor working with female victims.

Although our main purpose is to supply guidance for those working with adult women who have been raped, we believe it essential to provide some discussion of the treatment of the sexually abused child. The victimization of children is a subject that arouses horror and indignation. All too often, we are blind to indicators of abuse because we are reluctant to consider such a noxious possibility. Once abuse is detected, a common impulse is to remove the child from the home if the abuser is a parent or to blame the parents for neglect if the abuse occurred outside the home. Such reactions result in alienating the parents from the treatment process and compounding their own guilt and feelings of being out of control. Clinical experience indicates that the welfare of the child is inextricably bound up in helping the parents cope with the fact of sexual abuse. Treatment must be geared to the entire family.

In Chapter 13, Renee S. Tankenoff Brant presents an overview of the special issues involved in identifying abuse and treating the child victim in the emergency room. She defines a variety of behaviors, ranging from sexual misuse through molestation, rape, and incest, that may come to the attention of emergency room personnel. The signs and symptoms that indicate the possibility of abuse are described. Parental involvement is essential throughout the process of making an assessment and a treatment plan for the child victim.

When we initiated our rape crisis intervention program, we assumed that women would be superior to men in offering counseling to victims. But in order to ensure 24-hour coverage of our emergency room, we had to include men in our counseling roster. We found ourselves rather shame-faced about our brand of reverse sexism as we saw that the men could be as effective and empathetic as many of our female counselors. The majority of women victims responded positively to the male counselors, although there were some who felt comfortable sharing their feelings only with another woman. These wishes are respected in our assignment for follow-up. Warmth, empathy, concern, and skill are the most important qualities in the making of an effective counselor. Gender is secondary. Just as women need to be aware of their own feelings and reactions aroused by working with rape victims, men must also be prepared to cope with certain anxieties.

In Chapter 14, Daniel Silverman details the kind of preparation neces-sary for men to work with female victims of sexual assault. He emphasizes the stress and countertransference issues as well as the need for men to disabuse themselves of the misconceptions that abound about rape. Help-lessness, terror, and vulnerability are not emotions exclusively felt by women. Men can also come to understand the kind of trauma provoked by sexual assault and thereby add another dimension to the treatment of rape victims.

13

The Child Victim

Renee S. Tankenoff Brant

The sexual abuse of children includes many different kinds of behavior. One study has shown that only one-third of the reported cases involved rape or incest and that two-thirds involved *molestation,* which is defined as noncoital sexual contact (Sgroi, 1975). A *sexual assault* is nonconsensual manual, oral, or genital contact by the offender with the genitalia of the victim. *Incest* is coital contact between a blood relative and a child. *Rape* is defined, state by state, in the same way that it is for adult victims, but *statutory rape* is a special category of offense in which the law considers rape to have occurred, even though the victim may have consented, because the victim was younger than a legally defined "age of consent" (Breen, Greenwald, & Gregory, 1972).

Sexually assaultive behavior involving force and threats of force are obviously traumatic to the victim. However, sexual molestation, which may not involve force or intimidation, can be equally disruptive to a child's psychosexual development. This sort of trauma should also be treated seriously. Particularly in these less dramatic forms of abuse, adults dealing with children must be sensitive to the indirect ways in which the child may call attention to the problem and ask for help. Later in this chapter, the author describes some of these indirect signals that children may use.

In working with sexually abused children, the single most important fact to bear in mind is that the family, as well as the victim, must be included in any treatment program and is central to its success. Even in cases where parental neglect or abuse has not directly caused the problem, parents must participate in understanding the issues and in planning and

Renee S. Tankenoff Brant, M.D. ● Instructor in Psychiatry, Harvard Medical School; Director, Sexual Abuse Treatment Team, Children's Hospital Medical Center, Boston, Massachusetts.

carrying out the treatment program. The adequate resolution of their feelings about the incident is always important to the child's resolution:

> An 11-year-old girl was walking home from a skating rink along a familiar route in the daytime. A man in a parked car forced her into his vehicle and, under threat of violence, forced her to perform fellatio. Intercourse was attempted, but there was no penetration. The man then released the child, and she went home and told her parents. They immediately brought her to the emergency room. Initially the parents and the child appeared composed and controlled. Subsequently, the child developed some anxiety and mild phobic symptoms that soon abated, but the father reported that his wife had become acutely anxious and guilty. He feared that she was "falling apart." A short-term crisis intervention program for this family included individual work with the child but focused on the mother's acute response to the trauma.

Sometimes, parental concerns about rape can express the parents' anxiety, as opposed to any facts about the child's actual experience. The next case illustrates this:

> A psychiatrist was asked to see a 4-year-old girl, who was brought to the emergency room by her very anxious parents. She had been playing with a friend when a strange man walked up to them and asked directions to a nearby apartment. The 4-year-old was briefly left alone with the man while the friend left. Later, when the 4-year-old told her parents about the incident in a matter-of-fact manner, they brought her to the emergency room, fearful that she had been molested. Medical and psychiatric examination failed to reveal evidence of sexual misuse. The child was functioning well at home and at school. In follow-up visits with the parents, the psychiatrist discovered that both the father's sister and the mother of the child had been subjected to sexual misuse as children.

However, it also must be remembered that very often, it is the parent or the parent-substitute who has been the actual sexual offender with the child. One study showed this to be true in as many as 72% of the cases (DeFrancis, 1969). Also, while most attention is directed toward the male abuser and the female victim, there are also documented incidents of mother–son abuse as well as both male and female homosexual abuse.

In some of these familial situations, the circumstances are complex and subtle enough to warrant the term *sexual misuse* instead of *abuse*. In the following example, a parent certainly stopped short of abuse but still participated in increasing the child's anxiety and fantasies:

> A 7-year-old girl was brought to an emergency ward by her very concerned parents because she could not be disabused of the fantasy that she was pregnant. The child was referred for psychotherapy, and, in the course of this, it was discovered that her father occasionally drank.

At these times, his normal loving parental caresses became exaggerated. For the child, this raised vivid unconscious wishes and fantasies. Fact and fantasy became blurred, and her emotional experience was of incest, even though no genital contact had been made.

Sometimes mundane family routines or interactions might be sexually overstimulating to a child, even though the parent has not participated in any sexual event. A counselor can sometimes be helpful in determining and clarifying such a problem. In the following example, a mother was having trouble setting limits around bedtime, and the child interpreted this difficulty in a sexual way:

A 4-year-old male child was brought to the emergency ward because of increasing bedtime terrors. For six months, he had been increasingly insistent that his previously casual bedtime ritual with his mother be prolonged. At the point when the child was brought to the hospital, he was clinging to his mother for several hours each night before falling asleep, seeming to be in a panic and unable to let her leave. Play therapy with the child revealed his fantasy that his clinging to his mother was interfering in his parents' relationship, which indeed proved to be the case. The child's anxiety had arisen from the fact of his intense conflict between wanting to keep his mother for himself and feeling guilty and fearful about the selfishness and the destructiveness of his behavior to his parents' relationship.

Then, there are cases of direct, overt sexual abuse on the part of parents with their children:

A mother came to the emergency ward with her two daughters, ages 9 and 13. She had just discovered that her husband had been having regular sexual contact with the older child for seven years and with the younger one for two years. The older daughter's confession of this behavior to the mother was precipitated by the onset of her menses, at which time the mother talked with her daughter about reproduction and the daughter told her mother of the sexual contact between herself and her father.

In any event, the important first step toward the protection of children is the willingness of the counselor, and of other responsible adults, to recognize the possibility that sexual misuse or abuse can occur to children. Social taboos against sexuality between adults and children, and the anxiety generated in the adult by the recognition of violations of these taboos, seem to account for some misdiagnoses of children's somewhat disguised complaints to emergency wards:

An adult psychiatric patient in regular psychotherapy for episodes of acute anxiety revealed in her history that she had been regularly abused by her two teenage brothers, who threatened her if she told her parents.

When she complained to her mother of vaginal pain, she was consciously hoping that her mother would guess her problem and save her from her brothers' threats, as well as from further sexual exposure. The patient was taken by the mother on four separate occasions to a local emergency ward for these complaints and was sent away without even a physical exam. Neither the mother nor the doctors ever guessed.

The age of a child is usually important in making an assessment. In general, preadolescent children have difficulty verbalizing their problems and are frequently reluctant to approach people outside the family for help. They are more likely to come to medical settings with nonspecific symptoms or changes in their general functioning and adaptation. Symptom formation may differ with the age of a child. In latency-age children, younger than 9 or 10, nonspecific presenting symptoms may include hyperactivity, difficulty sleeping, fears, nightmares, phobias, overly compulsive behavior, and learning problems. Compulsive masturbation, precocious "sexual" play, and excessive curiosity about sexual matters are behavioral symptoms that may be more specific manifestations of sexual abuse.

The mother of a 7-year-old girl called the emergency psychiatrist after she learned that the child had been engaging in mutual masturbation with her maternal granduncle over a period of three months. This elderly man had lost his wife some months before, and the child had been spending some weekends with him to relieve his loneliness. During this time, the child became enuretic. The mother had noticed increased activity, sleeping problems, night fears, and an upsurge of sexual curiosity. The child's preexisting preoccupation with cleanliness assumed compulsive proportions. The mother finally learned about the child's experiences from a young aunt, in whom the child confided.

Sexually misused children can also complain of physical problems, such as pain on urination, genital laceration, abrasion, contusion, bleeding, irritation, infection, or genital discharge. Frequently, the history accompanying a case of genital injury indicates that the child fell in the bathtub or suffered some other accidental trauma. In cases of vulvar irritation, parents may blame bubble bath as the cause. While such histories and explanations may be true, it is important to entertain other possibilities. History taking must be tactful and should focus on the child's general behavior. It is helpful to assess parental anxiety and guilt as well as parent–child interaction. Follow-up in a nonthreatening setting is especially important in those cases where the examiner is uncertain of the etiology of the symptom. Some cases may require active outreach.

Venereal disease in children is being reported with increasing frequency and must be considered in any child presenting with genital discharge, irritation, or infection. In Maryland, a family-centered approach was used to screen for new cases of gonorrhea. In randomly selected families, 16% of the members had new cases of gonorrhea. Among the children, one-third were male. The average age of the child male patients was 7 to 10 years old, and the average age of the child female patients was 3 to 10 years old [Singer, unpublished (1975)]. Although some studies indicate that children may contract venereal disease as a consequence of poor hygiene and by other means than by direct contact, most studies of the transmission of venereal disease indicate that direct contact is most often the cause.

Children previously exposed to sexual misuse are also at high risk for repeated trauma. These children may provoke further misuse in an attempt to master the traumatic event. This is not to say that children are held responsible in these situations, as adults are always assumed to have and to exercise better judgment. It is likely that some especially severely neglected children receive some gratification in a close relationship with an adult, even though it involves sexual abuse of the child. The child may be unable to satisfy needs in other ways and may continue to seek pleasure, need satisfaction, or a masochistic experience of attention by provoking continued misuse. These children may present to emergency room settings with complaints of "rape," genital injury, or infection:

> A 5-year-old with vaginal bleeding and vulvovaginal irritation was brought to the emergency room by her mother. Included in the child's background were episodes of physical abuse in early infancy and a foster home placement in which the child was sexually abused by an adolescent. When the child was returned to her natural mother, she began visiting the house of her estranged father, and there she slept in the bedroom with 7- and 8-year-old sons of the father's girlfriend. The 5-year-old claimed that during the night, the boys stuck her genitals with pins. She told her father the next morning, but he did nothing. She repeated the story to her mother, who initially did not respond. The next day, the mother noted bloody spots on the child's underwear and took her to the emergency room. The child presented herself as a bright, precocious, seductive 5-year-old, who sat with her legs spread apart. She spoke of her boyfriends in school, whom she hugged and played with in the bathroom. She spoke with sadness of her father's absence from the family and of her anger toward her mother, who would not let her see father more often.

Adolescent pregnancy may also be a presenting symptom for sexual misuse. Inquiries should always be made into the circumstances leading to pregnancy. Often fear, guilt, and denial operating within adolescents and their families keep them away from clinics and emergency rooms. Only when pregnancy is suspected do these children come to medical attention.

The management of cases of child sexual misuse can be difficult. After determining as clearly as possible what has actually happened, the immediate physical and emotional needs of the child and the family must be addressed. Because of possible parental involvement in the assault, this can be a delicate procedure. However, sometimes the parent, having finally brought the child for care, is really asking for some help himself. With support and encouragement, these families can sometimes be helped to address the issue of sexual misuse directly.

In any event, the initial contact with misused children and families in emergency settings is crucial in determining whether the family will see professionals as helpful and worthy of trust or as unhelpful, judgmental intruders. In the latter case, return for follow-up is highly unlikely. Establishing a trusting alliance in the emergency setting makes subsequent therapeutic intervention possible. Thus, in all interactions with the child and the family, the important matter of building an alliance is primary.

Many medical centers have developed a team approach to deal with cases of sexual and physical misuse. Team members and consultants may include such varied professionals as pediatricians, nurses, gynecologists, child psychiatrists and psychologists, social workers, child-abuse specialists, and attorneys. Regardless of the makeup of the team, it is important that a clear plan be outlined and organized so as to avoid diffusion and redundancy.

It is important that the intervention itself be as atraumatic as possible. Hastily performed genital exams (Josselyn, 1962; Rothchild, 1967), insensitive questioning, and an upset and anxious emergency staff may contribute to feelings of anxiety, guilt, and shame. This sort of approach may be experienced as a form of attack by both the child and the family.

The clinical interviews with the child and the family should precede the physical exam unless a physical emergency is present. A very tactful and careful sorting out of fact, fantasy, and distortions in both child and parents is one of the most important yet most difficult tasks facing the examiner. Different family members sometimes present very different accounts. Especially when it is unclear what happened to the child, it can be helpful to interview family members separately. At all times, it is important to observe the nature of the feelings and the anxiety accompanying a person's story. These observations and feelings may be important in establishing the reality of a parent's or a child's story. Observations of interactions between various family members and behavior changes when they are together or alone can provide important, nonverbal data about the story. Whenever it is possible to corroborate stories presented by children or parents, this should be done.

The child and the family should be approached in a quiet, unrushed manner, with respect for their privacy. The child should be permitted to communicate his or her version of what happened. An attempt should be made to assess the acute emotional impact of the incident on the child and to assess the child's previous general adaptation and psychosexual development.

Some parents bringing their children for examination because of sexual trauma state that they would prefer not to have the child questioned about the event. They feel that it is better to "forget about it" and that by speaking to the child about the trauma, one will somehow make it worse. Such requests by parents are usually a reflection of their own anxiety and general sexual discomfort, if not specifically a fear of being found out. This tendency toward avoidance may be a characteristic style of handling upsetting events through denial. It is important to allow such parents to voice their concerns and anxieties. With support, they may be able to allow their children "permission" to talk. Many children may refuse to speak to examiners unless they sense that their parents feel it is all right. Parents should be informed that children are often tremendously relieved to be able to discuss these matters and that often they see the opportunity to do so as an indication of the parents' concern and love for them.

The parents must also understand that the professionals recognize, in the fact of their presence at a source of help, that the parent does care for his child. An attitude of understanding instead of blame is important to convey to the parents, also.

In general, a nonjudgmental approach aimed toward helping all family members is most profitable. The child and the family must all be viewed as patients. However, nonjudgmental does not necessarily mean nonauthoritarian. In many instances, reporting sexual abuse to the proper governmental agencies not only is legally mandated but can actually be seen as a caring and anxiety-reducing therapeutic measure. Parents are often frightened and guilty about their behavior and welcome even this intervention.

A basic differentiation must be made in the emergency ward between families that can be counted on to support and protect the child and families that may be too disorganized and disturbed to fulfill this function, even with therapeutic support. In cases where a child's safety and protection are in serious jeopardy, emergency room personnel may have to involve child welfare workers or take court action to protect a child. In extreme cases, this may involve removing the child from the home. Generally, this removal is temporary and is carried out together with a treatment plan for the family. The goal of this work is eventually to return the child to the family when that is feasible and in the child's best interests. Often, the hospital emergency room provides initial care and screening and then works with government agencies to develop a treatment program.

General physical examination should be performed before examination of the genitals. Complete genital examination is not always necessary. The examiner shoulds always attempt to explain to the child exactly what will be happening during the examination. Someone familiar to the child, usually a parent, should be present to comfort and to reassure the child. Indications for genital examination include complaints of pain, bleeding, and infection. The examination can be important also in reassuring the child of his or her intactness. Often external examination of the genitalia and aspiration of vaginal contents for the female child are sufficient, and a full internal examination is not needed.

Several articles have been written that describe in great detail the "ideal" medical–legal examination to be performed on sexually assaulted children (Capraro, 1967; Breen et al., 1972). While the accuracy of the reports of interviews and physical exam in the medical record is very important for possible legal use, some of these articles seem to suggest that the primary purpose of emergency intervention is to provide data for the legal system. In fact, in many cases, detailed genital examination is not indicated. The approach outlined by Lipton and Roth (1969) focuses on the physical and emotional care of children and their families as a primary concern, with legal concerns taking an important second place.

Before discharge from the emergency setting, it is important to have a meeting with the child and the family to summarize concerns, major findings, and plans for follow-up. Follow-up should be planned quite soon after the initial contact. Active collaboration between the therapeutic facility and protective services is often necessary. Preferably, one of the therapists involved in acute management of the case should continue with the family in follow-up. Goals of follow-up include further understanding and management of the acute situation, as well as following through on actualizing plans for longer-term intervention where indicated. In any event, but especially in situations where legal proceedings have been undertaken, important support can be provided by the emergency team for child and family to minimize the traumatic impact of the legal proceedings or of the transfer to a longer-term facility.

References

Breen, J., Greenwald, E., & Gregory, C. The molested young female: Evaluation and therapy of alleged rape. Pediatric Clinics of North America, 1972, 19(3), 717–725.

Capraro, V. Sexual assault of female children. Annals of the New York Academy of Science, 1967, 142, 817–819.

DeFrancis, V. Protecting the child victim of sex crimes committed by adults. Denver, Colo.: American Humane Association, 1969.

Josselyn, I. Psychological effect of the menarche. In W. S. Kroger (Ed.), Psychosomatic obstetrics, gynecology and endocrinology. Springfield, Ill.: Charles C Thomas, 1962.

Lipton. G. L., & Roth, E. Rape: A complex management problem in the pediatric emergency room. Journal of Pediatrics, 1969, 75(11), 859–866.

Rothchild, E. Anatomy is destiny. Pediatrics, 1967, 39, 532.

Sgroi, S. Molestation of children. The last frontier in child abuse. Children Today, 1975, 44(5–6), 19–24.

14

The Male Counselor and the Female Rape Victim

Daniel Silverman

Because rape represents a sexualized form of aggression directed most frequently against women, it is not surprising that female mental health professionals have assumed leadership both in studying the phenomena and in developing methods to assist victims in the posttraumatic period (Bassuk, Savitz, McCombie, & Pell, 1975). Clinical experience indicates that female rape victims may prefer to relate to women counselors during the acute phases of the crisis, perhaps because the victims assume that a woman can offer them empathy and understanding in this situation. However, the reality of crisis intervention work, whether carried out in the setting of the general hospital emergency ward, an acute psychiatric service unit, the local mental health center, or similar facilities, often dictates that male counselors, mental health workers, psychiatric residents, or physicians may be the first or only persons available to the female victims of rape. It is the purpose of this chapter to consider some of the possible difficulties inherent in being a male helping person assisting women in crisis following rape. It is hoped that these speculations will encourage others to share their impressions and experiences in this clinical area and that increased awareness of these problems may reduce the likelihood that they will interfere with potentially helpful intervention efforts.

Daniel Silverman, M.D. ● Instructor in Psychiatry, Harvard Medical School, Director of Medical Education, Department of Psychiatry, Beth Israel Hospital, Boston, Massachusetts.

This chapter has been adapted with permission from the *American Journal of Orthopsychiatry*, copyright 1977 by the American Orthopsychiatric Association, Inc., from "First Do No More Harm: Female Rape Victims and the Male Counselor," *American Journal of Orthopsychiatry*, 1977, 47(1), 91–96.

The first problem is the male counselor's response to the female victim, as he may find himself somewhat anxious at the prospect of being rejected by her in the initial meeting simply because he is a man. He may believe himself to symbolize the "masculinized" aggression from which the victim has suffered. The wish to somehow make up for the pain inflicted and to attempt to convince the patient that she need not fear all men may affect the counselor's approach. Feelings such as these could explain a pressure to make the intervention into a compensatory or corrective experience that will prove that some men can be gentle, empathic, and trustworthy. This attitude may also be the basis of changes in technique described by male psychiatric residents working in a rape crisis program. Modifications in strategy include changes in the use of space, physical contact, and tone of voice with the victim. Counselors speak more softly than usual; some increase physical distance from the women; others sit more closely; some hold the woman's hand or pat her shoulder; others feel that any such gestures would be inappropriate. The point to be made here is that if the male therapist is too anxious in attempting to reestablish the woman's capacity to trust a man, he may unknowingly offer either seductive or distancing nonverbal communications.

Another real possibility affecting the male counselor's response to the woman is that he may be subject to the same misconceptions about rape as the public at large. There is ever-increasing evidence that rape represents an act of extreme violence rather than sexual passion (Amir, 1971). At least in reported rapes, the crime has most often been perpetrated by young men, frequently in groups and in a premeditated fashion, against women of the same race, usually in their teens and 20s, although children and older women have been victimized as well (Amir, 1971). How misconceptions and biases may affect the counselor's ability to identify with the victim in an adaptive way is discussed below, but it must be said here that the counselor should examine his own understanding of what the crime of rape represents in terms of both victim and victimizer and familiarize himself with sociological and psychological studies on these subjects. Even more important, he should educate himself through open discussions with female colleagues about their presonal perceptions, experiences, and understanding of the topic. Review of videotaped and filmed interviews with rape victims may also offer useful perspectives.

Perhaps the most common error made by male counselors is to focus more on the sexual aspects of the rape than on the inherent violence. Such a focus can affect the empathic tone of the counselor's response. Many women describe their greatest concern during the actual trauma as fear for their lives. A woman sensing that her counselor fails to appreciate the intense violence she has suffered from may experience him as generally less supportive and less genuinely understanding.

A final factor that could influence the quality of the male counselor's interactions with the rape victim may be an unconscious wish to please the female directors, supervisors, or peers he is working with in the rape crisis intervention setting. There is a danger of being overly ingratiating or patronizing or of feeling pressured to prove to female associates and to the victim that his views and attitudes concerning rape and women's issues in general are as "liberal and liberated," "unchauvinistic," and "politically acceptable" as possible. Once again, overzealousness on the part of the counselor may offer the victim communications that she finds difficult to feel comfortable with or trust.

A second important issue is the male counselor's possible difficulty in empathizing with the female victim. Clinical experience indicates that generally female rape counselors find it easy to identify strongly with the woman rape victim. Although male counselors may be no less sensitive and caring than their female counterparts, they may have greater difficulty in identifying with the female victim. Male counselors may unconsciously identify not only with the victim but also with the rapist or the important males (husband, boyfriend, brother, or father) in the victim's life. Among the most common emotions experienced by the woman in response to rape trauma are tremendous feelings of helplessness and vulnerability. Counselor identification with the rapist could be an example of identification with the aggressor to defend against one's own feelings of helplessness and vulnerability aroused in trying to support the victim through her crisis. Such an identification may take the subtle forms of consistently questioning the victim's credibility and her degree of responsibility for the rape or of being concerned with the accused man's legal vulnerability because of "groundless allegations."

Strong identifications with the victim's boyfriend, husband, or father may take the form of a righteous indignation that the woman-as-an-extension-of-her-man has been raped and thus the man and all men have been violated. Attitudes of women as "man's property" have long-standing historical precedents in many cultures (Brownmiller, 1975) and may explain some male counselors' unconscious anger toward certain victims for "allowing the rape to happen." Identifications with the victim's mate may also be expressed as paternalistic overprotectiveness, a mechanism perhaps for assuaging feelings of guilt and responsibility for what has happened to the "defenseless" female victim. Overly patronizing attempts to rescue the victim from her environment or the aftermath of the rape are potentially counterproductive. Such gestures may communicate the message that the victim is indeed viewed as being helpless, thus increasing her own sense of vulnerability.

The unifying theme here is that allowing himself to identify with the victim may serve to attack the male counselor's sense of "this could never happen to me." Clearly, many women in our society have been forced by reality to see rape as a true possibility in their lives. Because it is comparatively rare for a man, in the general population, to be raped, it is much easier for men to maintain denial of anxiety about it. Throughout their lives, women have to confront feelings of vulnerability and helplessness in this society much more directly than men and may in general achieve greater mastery or acceptance of the attendant anxiety. This fact could offer a partial explanation of the female counselor's potentially greater comfort in assisting the rape victim in experiencing, containing, and tolerating her feelings of powerlessness and defenselessness.

While few male counselors working in nonpenal institutions have experience in dealing with male victims of rape, male counselors in a rape crisis intervention program often imagine that they would be more uncomfortable counseling male rape victims than female victims. In this case, the counselor might find it more difficult to deny feelings about being a victim himself. Unconscious conflicts about homosexual feelings could also be elicited in such situations, serving to further increase the counselor's uneasiness. The important point to be made here, whether one is counseling male or female victims, is that should the counselor's own anxieties cause him to retreat from dealing directly with the affects of the victim, he risks confirming the client's suspicion that what has occurred is so awful that it cannot be discussed.

A third area of importance is the female rape victim's response to the male counselor. A profound sense of helplessness coupled with powerful feelings of guilt and devaluation have been among the most universal of the early responses observed in female rape victims (Burgess & Holmstrom, 1973, 1974; Notman & Nadelson, 1976; Sutherland & Scherl, 1970). Clearly, these feelings may make the initiation of trusting relationships in the immediate posttraumatic period difficult. This problem could be heightened in the case of forming a new relationship with a man, because the woman's trauma was the result of masculine aggression. These facts must be kept in mind by the male counselor as he begins his interaction with the victim. She may be guarded in responding to overtures to enter an alliance, no matter how well meaning his intentions.

Another common feature of the victim's initial response pattern after rape is the displacement of anger. It may be extremely difficult for some women to express anger toward their assailant. The reasons may include fear of reprisal and a culturally determined inhibition of direct aggressive expression on the part of the woman. Redirection of the anger can occur and may be aimed at friends, family, police, or helping professionals. Women helpers may be spared, and men, including the counselor, may find themselves the objects of a hostility that is both puzzling and disheartening. Again, prior awareness of this possibility and an understanding of the sources of the anger may help the counselor to handle the affect in a nondefensive, nonpunitive way.

Finally, if the victim is seen in extended follow-up counseling, the full spectrum of feelings experienced by patients in various forms of therapy may be expected to emerge, including erotic responses directed toward the male counselor. Because of the extraordinary set of circumstances that bring client and counselor together in rape crisis, eroticized feelings may be experienced as more disquieting and anxiety-provoking for both client and counselor than under more usual therapy conditions. The increased impact of the emergence of erotic emotions in a setting where feelings of significant shame and humiliation have been shared may be dealt with more constructively by the male counselor if he is prepared for it. Sexual concerns in general commonly arise for the rape victim (Burgess & Holmstrom, 1973). Women with no sexual experience prior to the attack may be violently forced to confront sexual feelings without opportunity for any emotional preparation. A victim who has been active sexually may experience considerable anxiety about sex on resuming relations with her boyfriend or husband. She may see herself as damaged merchandise or fear accusations of infidelity. In other cases, she may express concern over future relationships with men, and this concern may have great relevance to her interactions with the male counselor. She may question her capacity to cope with men in general and may experience fears of being overwhelmed and then abandoned. The counselor's appreciation of the victim's heightened sensitivity should help him to reassure her that sexual feelings are natural, understandable, and common in people receiving professional counseling. The occurrence of such feelings in the counseling relationship provides the victim with the opportunity to understand and master accompanying anxieties that can interfere with her relationships with men. The counselor's acknowledgment that sexual feelings may be an area of concern indicates that such feeling can be openly addressed in an atmosphere of acceptance.

It is wise neither to except nor to ask for an immediate and firm commitment on the part of the victim for return visits or contacts. Telephone follow-up may be less invasive and allow the woman more safe distance and latitude in deciding about the future direction and intensity of counseling. While the counselor takes the initiative in offering follow-up contacts, the frequency and timing of the contacts should be decided by the client. Awareness of the victim's guardedness may help prevent the counselor from communicating a sense of personal disappointment or rejection that could heighten her feelings of guilt. The woman seeking professional help in the form of gynecological examination, crisis counseling, or legal advice may fear that the experience will revive a sense of the original trauma. The male counselor must prevent the intervention from becoming in any way a symbolic re-creation of the rape. Overzealousness and too forceful an attempt to convince the victim to accept help may be experienced as aggressive or assaultive communications. The victim's sensitivity in interpersonal relations must be given continuous consideration.

Of the conclusions that emerge from the preceding discussion, perhaps the single most important is that the crisis intervention should not be burdened with the primary goal of being a corrective or compensatory experience. An increasing understanding of the course of the posttraumatic syndrome following rape indicates that the reconstitutive process is a long-term phenomenon. Letting the patient know that the counselor is sensitive, aware of significant potential conflicts, and available when needed is as much as one should wish to communicate in initial encounters.

A male counselor has the responsibility to educate himself about the prevalent misconceptions about rape. He must examine his personal biases concerning this emotionally laden topic and recognize values, beliefs, and identifications that might interfere with communications of empathy to the victim. Open and ongoing exchanges with female colleagues may be extremely helpful in accomplishing this end.

The counselor must be both aware of and prepared for the sources of feelings that lessen the victim's capacity to trust others and to enter into new relationships. Such an awareness will help the counselor guard against his personalization of the victim's responses and could facilitate the working through of these feelings. Much care should be taken to prevent the counseling experience from becoming a recapitulation of the original trauma. Fantasies of rescuing the victim, the wish to please supervisors and colleagues, or fears of rejection may create performance pressures that can be translated into overaggressiveness on the part of the counselor and may be experienced by the woman as assaultive or confrontational and thus traumatic. The counselor must continuously consider his own feelings and their affect on his responses to the victim. Supervisory sessions or peer-group conferences of counselors are good places for such self-exploratory exercises.

References

Amir, M. *Patterns of forcible rape.* Chicago: University of Chicago Press, 1971.

Bassuk, E., Savitz, R., McCombie, S., & Pell, S. Organizing a rape crisis program in a general hospital. *Journal of the American Medical Women's Association, 1975, 30,* 486–490.

Brownmiller, S. *Against our will: Men, women and rape.* New York: Simon & Schuster, 1975.

Burgess, A. W., & Holmstrom, L. L. The rape victim in the emergency ward. *American Journal of Nursing, 1973, 73,* 1741–1745.

Burgess, A. W., & Holmstrom, L. L. Rape trauma syndrome, *American Journal of Psychiatry, 1974, 131,* 981–986.

Notman, M., & Nadelson, C. The rape victim: Psychodynamic considerations. *American Journal of Psychiatry, 1976, 133,* 408–412.

Sutherland, S., & Scherl, D. Patterns of response among victims of rape. *American Journal of Orthopsychiatry, 1970, 40,* 503–511.

VII

Appendixes

The following appendixes are based on protocols and forms developed by the Rape Crisis Intervention Program at Beth Israel Hospital, Boston, Massachusetts. The first five appendixes include guidelines, forms, and information directly used in victim care. Appendix 4 was prepared in conjunction with the Brookline Police Department. Appendix 5 addresses itself to the rape victim and is supplied to victims in the hospital emergency unit. Appendixes 6, 7, and 8 are examples of handouts used in community education programs. They have been developed to encourage discussion and provide necessary information about assault prevention and the medical, counseling, police, and court-related procedures and resources available to victims.

Guidelines for the Nursing Care of Rape Victims in the Emergency Unit

The emergency unit nurse is a key person in the team approach to the care of rape victims provided by the rape crisis intervention program. The nurse, the gynecologist, and the counselor coordinate their skills to provide sensitive and comprehensive treatment. The nurse is the first person to greet the rape patient and sets the tone for the patient's stay in the emergency unit. The nurse may be the only female member of the treatment team and the person with whom the patient may feel most comfortable. Concern for the patient's physical and emotional well-being should be actively demonstrated. Willingness and skill in listening, in identifying the patient's main concerns, in providing information about procedures, and in offering comfort and support are as important as attending to the patient's physical needs.

ARRIVAL OF RAPE VICTIM IN EMERGENCY UNIT

1. *Triage rape victims as a priority.* The rape victim should *not* be left in the waiting room but should be taken immediately to the interview room. If that is not available, she should be taken to a quiet room. Identifying data, insurance information, permission forms, etc., should be taken once she is provided with privacy.

2. *Assess chief complaints and orient victim to the emergency unit.* The nurse is to introduce herself to the patient and briefly assess her chief complaints. The nurse is to document this initial assessment in the medical record. The patient is to be told what services are available to her in the emergency room, including an explanation of the medical exam and the counseling services. It should be explained that all procedures are her choice as well as why they are in her best interest. Hospital policy is that the decision to report to the police is made by the patient. The nurse should ask if the patient wishes to contact any friends or family or if she wishes to notify the police and should offer assistance if patient so desires.

Every effort is made to avoid delays and leaving the patient alone. If friends, family, or a counselor from the local rape crisis center have come with the victim, the victim should be asked if she would like that person to sit with her until the hospital's counselor arrives.

COORDINATING THE TEAMING WITH THE COUNSELOR AND THE GYNECOLOGIST

1. *Linking patient with the counselor.* The counselor is to be called down first to meet with the rape patient *before* the medical workup whenever possible and appropriate (i.e., if wounds are minor). The counselor remains with the patient throughout her stay in the emergency room and is available to meet with family and friends.

The counselor should be called in *all cases* as a routine part of the procedure. When the counselor arrives, the nurse is to brief him/her about the patient and introduce them.

2. *Policies regarding the counseling services:*
   a. *If the patient refuses to talk with a counselor,* the nurse should plan to take a more active role in offering support and information. She should inform the patient that if

she changes her mind and wants follow-up counseling, she should call the program director.

b. *If the patient is accompanied by a counselor from the local rape crisis center,* the hospital counselor should still meet with the patient and consult with the outside counselor to plan follow-up. The patient has a choice about which program she wishes to use for follow-up counseling. For example, some choose to use the hospital for psychological counseling and the local rape crisis center for legal–police advocacy and support groups.

c. *If the patient has a psychotherapist,* the hospital counselor should still be called. The counselor offers acute support, contacts the patient's therapist, and offers to be available to the therapist as a consultant; that is, follow-up counseling is done by the ongoing psychotherapist in most cases.

d. *Follow-up counseling is available to all rape victims and should be actively encouraged.* Within 24–28 hours after the emergency unit visit, the patient is assigned to a rape crisis counselor (who may be a psychiatrist, a psychiatric social worker, or a psychologist) who will call the patient and arrange an appointment time. Rape patients may be offered up to 12 visits of crisis intervention. The first visit is free; all subsequent visits are on a sliding fee scale for those victims not covered by insurance or Medicaid. Family members, boyfriends, and husbands should also be encouraged to use the counseling service. If the patient needs to be seen beyond 12 sessions or if she is having severe difficulties, the counselor will refer her to the psychiatry outpatient clinic for ongoing psychotherapy.

e. *If a patient presents some months or years after a rape,* she is to be instructed to call the program director, who will arrange for counseling and evaluation. If indicated, she can be referred to the psychiatry clinic for long-term therapy.

3. *Linking the patient with the gynecologist.* The nurse and the counselor are to estimate how much time is needed for the patient to talk to the counselor before the medical exam. The patient's emotional state, her chief concerns, and her need for information and preparation should be the guide. The nurse is to call the gynecologist and coordinate the patient's needs with the physician's schedule. The nurse is to brief the gynecologist about the patient's chief concerns and emotional state and to introduce physician and patient.

THE HISTORY TAKING AND MEDICAL EXAMINATION

Please see "Guidelines for the Medical Care of Rape Victims" (Appendix 2) for a detailed description of the procedures.

1. *Nurse and gynecologist are to take particular care in explaining to the patient the purpose of the history taking and the examination, and her treatment options.*

Because of the emotional trauma sustained by the patient and common feelings of helplessness, vulnerability, and fear, it is very important to engage the patient in participating in her care to help restore her sense of control. The patient needs to know what to expect and the reasons questions are asked and procedures performed.

A detailed description of the reported rape should be taken down by the gynecologist in the patient's own words. There are two reasons for this: (1) the report is part of the patient's medical record and functions as fresh complaint should she decide to report the crime to the police and go to court; (2) details about force, threats, struggle, and sexual acts are needed to guide the exam to check for signs of trauma; details about setting (e.g., outdoors on wet grass, indoors on blue rug) are needed to check for corroborating physical evidence on clothing and body.

A medical history and gynecological history are needed in order to determine appropriate

treatment, especially in regard to pregnancy prevention and prophylactic treatment for venereal disease. The side effects of any medication are to be carefully explained. Options for
postcoital contraception, including the morning-after pill, insertion of an IUD, menstrual
extraction, and abortion, should be clearly presented with their attendent risks and advantages
to ensure that the patient can make an informed decision about what she feels is best for her.

    2. *The nurse and gynecologist are to collect and preserve physical evidence.*

        a. *Clothing,* particularly undergarments worn during the reported assault, should be
observed and described. The patient is to be instructed to save the clothing without
laundering or mending and to store it in a *paper* bag. (Plastic bags may promote
deterioration of secretions.) She should give this evidence to the police should she
report the crime.

        b. *Foreign matter* such as soil, splinters, and fibers should be observed, recorded, and
collected during the examination of the patient's entire body, including external and
internal genitalia. Specimens collected should be placed in a clean vial or glassine
envelope and labeled with the date, the time, the patient's name, the unit number,
and the body part that the specimen was taken from.

        c. *Pubic hair* should be combed and put in vial or glassine envelope and labeled as
above. Comparison sample of at least 10 hairs from the patient should be collected,
placed in separate container, and labeled.

        d. *Fingernail scrapings* should be collected, put in vial or envelope, and labeled. These
will be checked for foreign skin, blood, etc.

    The patient should give written permission so that foreign matter, pubic hair, and finger-
nail scrapings can be turned over to the police by the nurse or the gynecologist (see Appendix
3). The police officer receiving the specimens is to sign the record acknowledging receipt with
date and time. (The specimens are analyzed by the police crime lab.) If the patient has not
decided whether to report the crime to the police at the time of her emergency visit, she should
be instructed to save her clothing at home and told that specimens will be held seven days. At
the end of seven days, they will be destroyed because the hospital cannot take responsibility
for storage beyond that time. She should tell the police to retrieve the specimens immediately,
should she report the crime. These specimens are to be stored in the locked cabinet for seven
days.

    3. *Laboratory specimens analyzed in the hospital must be marked and stored properly.*
All slides are to be marked with a *diamond pencil* with *the patient's full name, unit number,
date, and time.* The nurse is to label the jars and other specimen containers with the same
information before leaving the examining room. Because of the need to ensure proper documentation for possible use in court, the nurse is to stamp all bacteriology, cytology, and serology
slips. During the day, the nurse is to take the specimens directly to the cytology lab. During
evenings and nights, they are to be locked in the cabinet with instructions posted on the outside
of the cabinet for the day-shift nurse to take them to the lab in the morning.

    Results of the wet mount for motile sperm and results of the acid phosphatase tests should
be immediately recorded in the medical record.

    4. *Complete and careful recording in the medical record is essential.* The sheet entitled
"Medical Protocol for Reported Rape" (see Appendix 2) should be used to record history and
findings. Additional sheets should be added as needed to accommodate the incident report.
This serves as a guideline for all procedures and should be *done in detail and legibly* as it may
well be subpoenaed by the court.

    No judgments or conclusions are to be made in the record. It functions to document
observations and what the patient reports. "Reported rape" should be the phrase used in all
records, rather than "alleged rape," which carries a connotation of doubt or "the rape," which
is weighed in the other direction.

    It is imperative that hospital staff recognize that their task is to offer treatment and record
findings, *not* to make judgments about the patient's story. This is the job of the judge and jury.

The nurse is to check this protocol for completeness and accuracy; she should add any information she may have that is not recorded by the physician. Both nurse and physician sign the record.

Facilitating the Liaison between the Police, the Patient, and the Hospital

As stated above, it is up to the patient to report the rape to the police. Hospital policy is to encourage the patient to do so and to support her efforts to cooperate with the police investigation.

If the police accompany the patient to the emergency unit, the nurse should tell the officer approximately how long the patient will be involved with the gynecologist and the counselor so that the officer can plan for when he can talk with the patient and bring her home, if necessary. The officer will need to know how the patient is feeling and when would be the best time to speak with her. This is the patient's decision. The nurse may ask the patient if she wishes the nurse to stay while she talks to the officer. The officer is the best source to answer the patient's questions about the investigation procedures, concerns about safety, and court-related concerns. The nurse should encourage the patient to talk with the officer about these matters.

In order for the hospital to release information and specimens to the police, written permission from the patient must be obtained. There is a special consent form available in the emergency unit. It contains the patient's consent and an acknowledgment of receipt of physical evidence to be signed by the police officer. This form is to be kept in the medical record. The nurse is to explain to both the patient and the police officer that such permission is needed to protect rights of confidentiality.

Whenever possible, the patient's permission for release of physical evidence (clothing, fingernail scrapings, pubic hair, etc.) to the police crime lab should be obtained while she is in the emergency unit. Even if she delays several days before going to the police, the signed consent form will be in her record to avoid delay once she has reported. Because these specimens can be stored in the hospital only seven days, the patient should be encouraged to go forward within this time and to inform the police to immediately retrieve the items. The officer collecting these specimens must sign the form in the medical record with the date and time, and the nurse should sign as a witness.

If the patient has decided *not* to report the rape to the police, she should be encouraged to file an anonymous third-party report (see Appendix 4). Forms for this are in the emergency unit or can be obtained from the counselor the patient uses for follow-up. The completed third-party reports should be sent to the program director's office. The director is responsible for forwarding the reports to the proper police district. The patient should understand that no arrest can be made on the basis of this report.

Follow-Up Planning with the Hospital Team

The nurse is to make sure that the gynecologist gives the patient a follow-up medical visit to his/her clinic in six weeks. Before the patient leaves the emergency unit, the nurse is to check that the patient understands why and when her medical appointment is scheduled. The nurse is to review briefly with the patient any instructions about treatment or medication and to make sure that side effects are understood.

The nurse is to check with the counselor about the patient's plans for counseling follow-up. If the patient is to be followed at the hospital, the counselor and the nurse are to see that she understands that a follow-up counselor will be calling her within 24–48 hours to arrange an appointment.

The nurse and the counselor should make sure that the patient has transportation home and a safe place to stay. The police will provide a ride home; another resource is the local rape crisis center. If their services are needed, call ahead to avoid keeping either them or the patient waiting unnecessarily. If temporary shelter is needed, there is a list of resources in the emergency room.

Give the patient a copy of the information for patients coping with sexual assault (Appendix 5) before she leaves the emergency unit. It outlines steps in police and court procedures and gives resources.

Nursing staff should see the acting nursing liaison to the rape crisis intervention program if there are questions regarding the nursing care and emergency unit procedures with rape patients. Questions regarding medical care and procedures should be directed to the acting gynecology liaison. The director of the program should be consulted about counseling procedures and overall policy questions and problems.

Guidelines for the Medical Care of Rape Victims

PURPOSE

1. Diagnosis and treatment of trauma
2. Collection and documentation of medical evidence
3. Examination and prophylaxis for venereal disease
4. Evaluation and prophylaxis for pregnancy
5. Crisis intervention for emotional support

It is hospital policy to triage rape victims as a priority in the emergency unit even when there is no evidence of severe physical trauma. A team approach is required to provide sensitive and comprehensive care. The nurse, gynecologist, and counselor coordinate their skills and expertise to meet the multiple needs of the rape patient.

LEGAL ISSUES

In Massachusetts, the crime of rape is defined by law as sexual intercourse or unnatural sexual intercourse (i.e., fellatio, sodomy, or the penetration of any body orifice by a body part or object), performed without consent and with the use *or* threat of force. This means any person, male or female, can under law be the victim of rape.

Penetration and the use or threat of force are two critical legal elements which must be proven. The medical examination is key in providing corroborating evidence. The presence of sperm or semen, or trauma to external or internal genitalia are used to prove penetration. If force were used, signs of physical trauma would be expected but if *threat* of force were used, then there would not be observable trauma.

Because the rape patient is the victim of a violent crime, her examination involves an interface between the medical and legal professions. Detailed, legible, and complete documentation of physical observations and findings is essential. The Medical Protocol (see the end of this appendix) will aid this process. *Clear, readable, and comprehensive recording is necessary, since the medical record will be subpoenaed to court if the case is brought to trial.* The physician's observations of signs of penetration and force, the recording of the victim's account of the incident, and the integrity of the laboratory results are crucial elements in the court case.

A patient reporting rape or attempted rape should be urged to have a medical examination in her best interest. However, it is not mandatory and the decision is entirely hers.

All rape patients should be encouraged to report the crime to the police. Again, it is the patient's choice and responsibility to do so, and the hospital will provide her with care and support regardless of her decision. Should she decide not to go to the police, the option of anonymous third-party reporting should be explained to her.

History and Review of Symptoms

1. History of the assault incident. A detailed history of the assault events is to be taken by the physician and recorded in the patient's medical chart using the patient's own words. The nurse or the counselor is to be present to provide emotional support and to act as a witness. The assault history should include:

   a. Date, time, and location of the assault.
   b. Description of any threats, weapons, physical contact, restraints, violence, and any resistance by the patient.
   c. Description of any sexual acts attempted or completed. Include oral and rectal penetrations, as well as vaginal penetration, whether assailant ejaculated, use of a condom, use of foreign objects or instruments, and other degrading acts, e.g., being urinated upon.
   d. Description of any activity of the victim since the assault which would alter physical evidence, i.e., douched, bathed, inserted tampon or contraceptive jelly, changed clothes.

For those patients who have not yet gone to the police or who have not yet given them a detailed account of the assault, also include:

   e. How assailant gained access to victim; a description of the assailant(s), particularly any distinguishing characteristics (e.g., scars); how assailant left scene; and any statements made by the assailant. Record the exact words used. (Rapists characteristically use the same words and behavior repeatedly. This modus operandi is important in identifying possible suspects.)

2. General medical history
   a. Obtain history of allergies, medications, and major illnesses—including migraine, hypertension, seizures, venous disease, coagulation defects, a stroke, etc.—in order to evaluate appropriate treatment options.
   b. Obtain gynecological history of menses, last menstrual period, contraceptives, and infections in order to evaluate postcoital contraceptive options.
   c. Obtain statement of any current physical complaints.

The Physical Examination

1. Describe the patient's emotional state; note both your own observations (e.g., victim crying, trembling, withdrawn) and the victim's subjective report (e.g., "I feel afraid, helpless.")
2. Describe the condition of clothing worn during the assault; note any rips, blood or semen stains, mud, soil, or other foreign matter.

   a. *If police accompanied the patient* and are prepared to receive evidence, ask the victim's permission to collect her clothing (see Permission for Release of Evidence). Carefully place each item of clothing in a separate *paper* bag (plastic will promote deterioration of secretions). Do *not* fold across any stains. Label each bag with the patient's name, the unit number, the date and time of assault, and the piece of clothing contained, with a description of foreign matter observed and its location. Give the bags to the police and have the officer sign the receipt on the permission form. This form is then entered into the patient's medical record.

b. *If the patient has not reported the rape to the police* or is not wearing the clothing she had on at the time of the assault, instruct her to preserve the clothing herself in the above manner and to give it to the police if and when she should decide to report it. Encourage her to preserve the clothing even if she is doubtful about reporting since she may change her mind and valuable evidence will be lost unless she takes these steps. *Note:* This hospital cannot take responsibility for storing clothing.[1]

3. Examine the patient's entire body, including the external genitalia, for signs of trauma. Record location and describe exact appearance and size. Include bruises, lacerations, bleeding, fractures, etc. Use figure on Medical Protocol to illustrate location. The history of the assault is used to guide the examination of specific areas.

4. Examine the patient's entire body, including the external genitalia, for evidence of seminal fluid, foreign pubic hair, and foreign matter such as mud, splinters, fibers, etc.

a. *If genital contact occurred,* gently comb pubic hair for hairs transferred from assailant to victim. Use a clean comb available in examining room; place the hair, foreign matter, and comb in clean envelope, seal and label with patient's name, unit number, date and time of collection, date and time of assault, and description of contents. Then take a minimum of ten pubic hairs from the patient as a comparison sample. This may be done by a vigorous combing or plucking. It is critical to have at least three hairs with follicles. Place the second comb and hairs in a separate envelope, label as above, and indicate contents as patient's pubic hair sample.

b. *If any foreign matter is located,* collect, place in separate envelopes, and label as above. Include the location of matter when labeling (e.g., sand found in vagina).

c. *If the patient scratched the assailant,* take scrapings of her fingernails for traces of blood and tissue. Carefully scrape under each nail (avoid contaminating evidence with victim's blood by pricking her), place scrapings from each individual nail in a separate envelope or vial, and label as above, including which finger from which hand.

Note: These items of physical evidence will be stored by the hospital for retrieval by the police for analysis at the police crime laboratory. The patient's permission is needed on Permission for Release of Evidence. If police are present, this evidence should be transferred directly with the proper receipt. If the patient has not reported the rape to the police, encourage her to permit collection for evidence preservation, should she change her mind. Instruct her to tell the police to retrieve this evidence from the emergency room if and when she reports the crime.[2]

5. Examine internal genitalia for signs of trauma and seminal fluid. The pelvic exam is to be done with a *nonlubricated, water-moistened speculum to collect all laboratory specimens.* If appropriate, examinations of urethra, rectum, and pharyngeal cavity are to be performed. Once the laboratory specimens are collected, a bimanual examination is performed. Carefully record any evidence of trauma.

THE LABORATORY SPECIMENS

The laboratory specimens are to be obtained by the examining physician in the presence of a witness (the emergency unit nurse and/or counselor). The slides are to be carefully labeled

---

[1]Hospitals should state their policy regarding the storage of clothing.
[2]Hospitals should state their policy regarding the storage and transfer of material evidence to the police for analysis by the police crime laboratory.

with a diamond pen with the patient's name, the unit number, and the date of collection. The slides should *not* be put in the routine collection box. Between 8:30 A.M. and 5:00 P.M., the nurse is to personally deliver the slides to pathology. At night, store the slides in the locked cabinet with a note on the outside of the box to alert the day-shift nurse to hand deliver them to the pathologist. *Be sure to indicate on all cytology slips that the specimens are for reported rape so that the pathologist properly processes them.*

The following specimens are to be taken.

1. *Wet mount for motile sperm.* Specimens should be obtained from the vagina, cervix, and vulva. A drop of saline and a cover slip are placed on the slides to keep them moist. They are to be examined immediately by the physician and the results carefully recorded. If this is not possible, swabs should be placed in separate tubes with a saline solution.

2. *Acid phosphatase for seminal fluid.* Diagnostic tablets or tape are available in the emergency unit; directions are in the packet. Fluid may be aspirated from the vagina or rectum or oral cavity and tested immediately with the tablets or tape. Record the results. If this cannot be done immediately, all aspirated fluid should be stored in a labeled, screw-top jar and frozen. (Acid phosphatase is detectable up to six months postcontact.) Items of clothing or areas of dried semen on the skin are tested by touching those areas with a saline-moistened swab or filter paper for 15 seconds; the swab or paper is then tested for acid phosphatase.

3. *Culture and sensitivity for gonorrhea.* Specimens should be taken from appropriate areas, i.e., cervix, rectum, pharynx, and placed on Thayer-Martin plates. Take specimens to the bacteriology lab for incubation immediately. (Gonorrhea can be detected by culture within two hours after contact.)

4. *Baseline serological test for syphilis.* RPR, Hinton, or VDRL is taken. (Incubation for syphilis is 9–90 days.)

5. *Pap smears for the detection of sperm.* (These will also show cancerous cells, herpes, yeast, or trichomonas.) Samples should be taken from the endocervix, exocervix, and posterior fornix. Place on glass slides, label properly, and drop in Pap fixative bottle. Do not allow slides to dry in air.

Treatment of the Victim

1. *Treat all injuries.*
2. *Prophylactic treatment for venereal disease.* The options are

   a. Procaine penicillin 4.8 million units IM (intramuscularly), plus 1 gram of oral Benemid given simultaneously. (This is effective for most strains of gonorrhea and incubating syphilis.)
   b. Tetracycline 0.5 gram by mouth every 6 hours for 5 days. (Give this to patients who are sensitive to penicillin or who have an aversion to injection. It is effective for most strains of gonorrhea; 12-day course is effective for incubating syphilis.)
   c. Minocycline 50 milligrams by mouth 4 times daily for 5 days. (This is given to patients who are sensitive to penicillin and who wish to avoid gastrointestinal side effects of tetracycline. It is expensive.)
   d. Spectomycin 2 grams IM in a single dose. (It is not effective for throat gonorrhea, and its efficacy for incubating syphilis has not been established.)

3. *The risk of pregnancy must be assessed and postcoital contraception options explored.* A detailed menstrual history and the date of the patient's last menstrual period are needed to estimate risk of pregnancy.

a. *If the patient had an IUD in place at the time of the rape or is taking birth control pills,* she should be considered protected against pregnancy.

b. *If the patient is mid-cycle at the time of the rape and unprotected,* the following options may be considered:

  i. Postcoital insertion of an IUD may be offered within 48 hours of the rape. The effectiveness of this method is not well established. Risks and side effects are to be fully explained.

  ii. Menstrual extraction may be offered within two weeks of the missed period. Risks and side effects are to be fully explained. This option requires that the patient is willing to wait, tolerate uncertainty, and return for the procedure.

  iii. Therapeutic abortion (D & C) may be offered should her pregnancy test prove positive. She may return for a standard urine pregnancy test six weeks after her last menstrual period. Another option is to have a Beta Subunit (assay for human chorionic gonadotropin) drawn. It can determine pregnancy after 3 days of gestation, but, for maximum accuracy, 8 days should elapse after the rape. Beta Subunit should be used particularly if the patient is very distraught about the possibility of pregnancy and is mid-cycle. She should be informed about the expense of this test.

  iv. *Postcoital contraception medication.* At the present time, there is no FDA (Federal Drug Administration) approved medication for this purpose. Since the incidence of pregnancy after one unprotected intercourse is only between 1 and 5%, the possibility of pregnancy should be downplayed to decrease the victim's anxiety, and assurances should be given about the alternatives should pregnancy occur. Physicians may, at their discretion, choose to offer one of the following hormone treatments *only if* the patient is informed that the FDA does not approve this use of the medication and is given a full explanation of all risks and side effects. Side effects include nausea, vomiting, breast tenderness, delayed menses, remaining small chance of pregnancy, and higher ectopic rate should she be pregnant. If DES (diethylstilbestrol) fails to prevent pregnancy, then a therapeutic abortion should be performed since there is a probable risk to the fetus. The possibility of a prerape, desired pregnancy should be carefully ruled out before postcoital hormone treatment is given. The following medications may be used: diethylstilbestrol, 25 mg. po. b.i.d. ×5 days; ethinylestradiol, 5 mg. po. b.i.d. ×5 days; Premarin, 25 mg. IV daily ×3 days; Premarin, 50 mg. IV daily ×2 days. Use with Compazine, 10 mg. b.i.d. given simultaneously to decrease discomfort from side effects.

Medical Follow-Up

The patient is to be given a six-week follow-up appointment, in the Gynecology Clinic with the physician who treated her in the emergency unit. At that time, the patient should be examined and reassured as to her physical condition. She should be encouraged to take advantage of the counseling services of the hospital's rape crisis intervention program. If she is not seeing a counselor and wishes to see one at this time, a referral can be made by calling the program director.

The following lab work should be done at the 6-week follow-up visit:

  a. Cervical cultures and sensitivities.
  b. Repeat of the serologic test for syphilis.
  c. Pregnancy test, if appropriate.
  d. Blood typing, if requested for legal purposes.

Emotional Support and Follow-Up

The hospital's rape crisis intervention program provides rape crisis counselors who are on call 24 hours a day, 7 days a week, to the emergency room. The counselors are psychiatrists, social workers, and psychologists who are available to provide follow-up and referral as well as acute care for the rape victim. The counselors are also available for family members and friends of the victim.

When a victim presents in the emergency room, a rape counselor is immediately called. The counselor will usually meet with the patient before she is examined by the gynecologist and will be available to consult with the gynecologist. The counselor will provide the following:

1. Emotional support and psychological counseling for the victim, family members and friends.
2. Assessment of the crisis and the patient's coping resources.
3. Basic information about medical, legal, and psychological concerns.
4. Consultation to the medical staff and police.
5. Arrangements for follow-up counseling within 48 hours after the initial emergency-unit visit.

If there are any questions or comments regarding these guidelines, contact the program director or the gynecology liaison to the rape crisis intervention program.

MEDICAL PROTOCOL FOR REPORTED RAPE	
Time and date of arrival in E.R.	Patient's name: Address: Unit number: Birthdate:
Time and date of examination	
Time and date of reported rape	

Incident Report   (In patient's words - attach additional sheet if necessary; include time, place, circumstances, violence, threats, sex acts, etc.)

Signature (if not examining M.D.) Position

Medical History

Emotional State   (describe)

(continued)

Physical Examination   (Include all signs of external trauma and appearance of patient;
                         note details, such as torn clothing, broken fingernails, etc.)

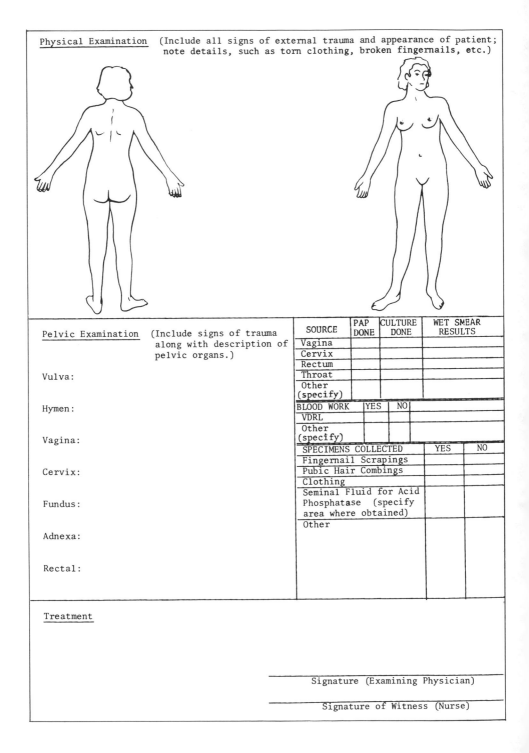

Pelvic Examination (Include signs of trauma	SOURCE	PAP DONE	CULTURE DONE	WET SMEAR RESULTS	
along with description of pelvic organs.)	Vagina				
	Cervix				
	Rectum				
Vulva:	Throat				
	Other (specify)				
Hymen:	BLOOD WORK	YES	NO		
	VDRL				
Vagina:	Other (specify)				
	SPECIMENS COLLECTED			YES	NO
	Fingernail Scrapings				
Cervix:	Pubic Hair Combings				
	Clothing				
Fundus:	Seminal Fluid for Acid Phosphatase (specify area where obtained)				
Adnexa:	Other				
Rectal:					

Treatment

_____
                        Signature (Examining Physician)

_____
                        Signature of Witness (Nurse)

Permission for Release of Material Evidence to the Police

I hereby authorize the hospital and its agents to supply the police with specimens of physical evidence to be analyzed by the police crime laboratory. This release will occur *only if I decide to report the incident to the police.*

These items include:

(check if appropriate items)

☐ fingernails scrapings
☐ foreign matter (specify): _____
☐ pubic hair combings and sample
☐ clothing (specify): _____

I understand that the above items of physical evidence will be held by the Hospital for 7 days following my examination and treatment in the emergency unit.[1] If I have not reported the incident to the police and instructed the police to collect this material within this time period, the hospital will destroy the specimens after 7 days since the hospital cannot take responsibility for storage beyond this time.

I understand that it is my decision and responsibility to report the incident to the police and to inform the police of the existence of the material evidence.

_____   _____
Date   Patient's Signature or Guardian's

_____   _____
Time   Witness's Signature

Acknowledgment of receipt of material evidence by the police

I hereby acknowledge receipt from the hospital of the following specimens of physical evidence checked above.

_____   _____
Officer's Police District   Police Officer's Signature

_____   _____
Time   Date   Witness's Signature

(Note: Attach this form to the packet of physical evidence. When the evidence is collected and the form is signed by the police, put form in patient's medical record.)

_____

[1]Hospitals should include their own policy regarding the storage of material evidence.

Third-Party Rape Report

The purpose of this form is to assist the police in identifying rapists when a victim does not want to report the rape to the police. There will be no effort by the police to identify the victim, and she will remain anonymous.

Date of attack: Time:

Location of attack (approximate):

_____

Description of rapist

Race   Age   Height   Weight   Build

Eye color   Hair color   Length of hair

Hairstyle   Mustache?   Beard?

Glasses?

Clothing

_____

Distinguishing characteristics (scars, speech peculiarities, etc.)

_____

Was vehicle used? (Describe) Reg. #   State

_____

If victim knows culprit, name and address:

_____

Description of attack (include circumstances, how first approached, sexual details, threats and force used, how culprit left; all statements and behavior of culprit are very important to describe). Attach additional sheets if necessary.

Information for Patients Coping with Sexual Assault

Because of the expected period of disruption, confusion, and upset that follows a major stress, the hospital offers special services to patients through the rape crisis intervention program. These services include:

In the Emergency Room:
1. Medical care for internal and external injuries, preventive treatment for venereal disease and pregnancy.
2. Acute crisis intervention by trained mental health professionals to give support, information, and assistance with immediate concerns.
3. Documentation of the facts of the assault and collection and preservation of physical evidence for possible use in police investigation and court.

Follow-Up Services:
4. Medical examination in our gynecology clinic *six weeks* after the initial visit to make sure treatment is effective. You should receive an appointment slip for the follow-up visit before you leave the emergency room.
5. Up to 12 sessions of crisis counseling to help with emotional reactions. You will be called within 48 hours after the emergency room visit by a crisis counselor. Counseling is also available to parents, husbands, and boyfriends.
6. Counselors are prepared to answer questions about police and court procedures.
7. Consultation on specific rape-related issues for the therapists of patients already in treatment elsewhere.
8. Availability of long-term psychotherapy and comprehensive psychiatric care when indicated.

The following information is given to answer some of the many practical questions people have about hospital, police, and court procedures. We hope this may help you with some of your concerns.

1. What is the cost of hospital services?
The emergency room and follow-up services are covered by insurance and Medicaid. If you do not have third-party coverage, fees will be adjusted along a sliding scale based on your financial resources. If you have no money at all, the hospital will provide services free under the Hill-Burton Act.

You are also eligible to apply to the state for reimbursement of treatment costs under the *Victims of Violent Crime Compensation Act* for expenses exceeding $100.00. Pamphlets describing this Act are available in the emergency room or from your counselor, or you may call the Bureau of Public Information in the Department of the Attorney General.[1]

---

[1] Include only in those areas of the country where applicable. Hospitals should investigate whether similar resources are provided by their municipal, county, or state governments.

2. Will the hospital automatically report the rape to the police?

No. Our policy is that it is your decision and responsibility. We will support what you feel is the best choice for you.

In this state, every police department has officers trained specially in rape investigation.[2] Our emergency room nurses and crisis counselors can tell you how to contact these officers in our area. If you want more detailed information before making a decision, our staff can refer you to special counselors attached to the court system. Talking to them does not obligate you to report to the police. It you should report, these specialists will go with you to the police and guide you through the court process.

3. What should I do with clothing I had on at the time of the assault?

You should *save everything,* without laundering or mending or altering it in any way. Place each item in a separate *paper* bag and give it to the police, who will check it over carefully in their crime lab for any physical evidence. Even if you are unsure about going to the police now, you should save the clothing just in case you change your mind.

4. What will the hospital do with the evidence it has collected?

Slides taken of secretions and sperm will be analyzed in our lab and recorded in your medical record. Your story told to the physician is also written in your medical record, as are the results of the physical examination. With your *written permission,* these can be made available to police. Should your assailant be arrested, your medical record will be subpoenaed by the court and presented as evidence.

Physical evidence such as fingernail scrapings, pubic hair samples, and foreign matter found on your body will be held by the hospital *for seven days* following your examination. We cannot take responsibility for storage beyond this time. If you report the assault to the police in the next few days, you must tell them to come immediately to the hospital to collect this evidence. We cannot release these items without your written permission. We recommend that you sign a release form now so that delays can be avoided. This gives the hospital permission to release this evidence to the police *if* you report the rape to the police, and if you tell them to come here.

5. Is there anything else I can do to prepare for going to the police or testifying in court?

Yes, it is a good idea to write down your account of the assault. Some people recall everything right away and then later have trouble remembering. Others recall details days afterward that initially were forgotten. We recommend that you write down your own account for yourself. *Remember to add to it if things come to mind later.* Be as detailed and complete as possible about exactly what was said and done. Include how you were approached, all conversation even if it seems trivial, threats, weapons, time, place, description of the assailant, his behavior, your behavior, what was demanded and what was performed. Include the physical–sexual details even though these may be difficult to think about and write. The reason for details is that individual assailants usually have characteristic patterns in what they say, demand, and do. Your account may help the investigator identify a suspect and will assist you and the prosecuting attorney in preparing for trial.

---

[2]Include only in those areas of the country where applicable. In Massachusetts, every police department in the state is required by law to have officers trained in rape investigation. Hospitals should inquire about similar laws or practices in their communities.

6. *If I don't want to talk to the police or go to court, is there anything else I can do?*

Yes. If you definitely decide that you do not want to report the rape to police, you may submit *an anonymous third-party report*. This report includes a description of the assailant and the assault much the same as described above in number 5. It has the advantage of alerting the police to the danger in the community, and your description may help with other cases under investigation. It has the disadvantage that no arrest can be made on the basis of a third-party report even if they have a suspect, since a complaining witness is needed. The third-party report forms are available from our emergency room nurses and from your crisis counselor. The staff will be responsible for getting the information to the proper police authorities.

7. *Is it true that the court can require me to answer questions about my prior sex life?*

Not any longer.[3] In the spring of 1977, a law was passed that says that a person's prior sexual conduct cannot be admitted as evidence in court except under two specific conditions:

a. if the prior sexual behavior occurred with the defendant.
b. if the sexual behavior was recent enough to explain any physical evidence that was found (for example, the presence of sperm could be accounted for by the fact that the woman had intercourse with her husband four hours before the reported rape).

8. *Do I need to hire a lawyer if I plan to take the assailant to court?*

No. Rape is a serious felony and comes under criminal law. The state always brings charges against the defendant in a rape case. Your role is that of a witness for the prosecution. A prosecuting attorney (the district attorney, or DA) will be assigned to your case. He or she will prepare you to testify in court. Ask questions about what concerns you and remember that the better prepared you are, the easier it will be for you in court. Poor preparation will seriously hinder the state's case against your assailant.

9. *What are the steps in the court process?*

Most cases go through three stages in the criminal justice system:

a. *Probable cause hearing.* You, the DA, a police officer (usually the detective assigned to your case), other witnesses, the defendant, and his lawyer are present. You will be asked to testify and also will be questioned by the defendant's lawyer. The defendant probably will not testify, and the judge (there is no jury) will decide whether there is enough evidence to refer the case to the grand jury.
b. *Grand jury.* Just you, the DA, other witnesses, and the police detective appear before a jury of 24 persons. This is a closed hearing. Neither the defendant nor his lawyer is present. The grand jury decides whether or not to indict the defendant. If an indictment is returned, then the case is referred to the superior court for trial.
c. *Superior court.* The full trial, usually with a jury (the defendant has the choice of a judge or a judge and jury), occurs here. You, other witnesses, the detective, lawyers for the prosecution and for the defense, and the defendant are present. There is presentation of testimony and evidence with cross-examination. A verdict is reached here, and if the defendant is convicted, he will be sentenced by the judge who conducted the trial.

---

[3]Laws vary from state to state. Hospitals should be familiar with the laws in their states which pertain to rape and the rules of evidence in rape cases. This information should be provided to the rape patient.

We have not attempted to anticipate questions you may have about your medical care or emotional well-being. Worries and concerns are common. It takes time to recover from a major stress like sexual assault. Please talk with our emergency room staff and counselors. They are here to help you.

	Phone Numbers
Emergency Room	
Gynecology Clinic	
Director, Rape Crisis Intervention Program	

Rape Questionnaire

These statements reflect common ideas about rape. Please respond honestly (True or False) to the following:

	T	F
1. Rape is almost exclusively an inner city phenomenon.	___	___
2. Rapists are usually men deprived of sexual relations.	___	___
3. Most children who are raped know their assailants.	___	___
4. If there is no weapon or actual physical violence a woman cannot bring charges of rape.	___	___
5. It is common for more than a year to pass before a rape case comes to trial.	___	___
6. Women who hitchhike or go alone to bars are asking to be raped.	___	___
7. Hospitals will automatically notify the police and the victim's family.	___	___
8. In the majority of rape cases the victim and assailant are of different races.	___	___
9. A wife can be raped by her husband.	___	___
10. Immediately after a rape, some women are very composed and calm.	___	___
11. Being raped ruins a woman's future sexual adjustment.	___	___
12. Every police department in Massachusetts is required by law to have officers trained in rape investigation.	___	___
13. Many rapes would be eliminated if women would not dress seductively.	___	___

The Rape Questionnaire covers commonly misunderstood myths and facts concerning rape. It is designed as an educational tool to promote discussion. Participants are asked to fill out the questionnaire at the beginning of an educational program. The review of the questions and responses usually leads to lively exchanges and rapid identification of some of the sociocultural, psychological, medical, and legal issues that need clarification. This questionnaire is not intended to serve as a research instrument.

	T	F

14. In order to press charges, the victim must hire an attorney. ___ ___

15. Most women who are raped blame themselves. ___ ___

16. Testimony about the woman's past sexual conduct is important evidence in a rape trial. ___ ___

17. Many victims do not tell their husbands, parents or family that they were raped. ___ ___

18. It is unnecessary for a victim to go to a hospital unless there is physical injury. ___ ___

19. Rapists often know their victims. ___ ___

20. Rape victims are frequently rejected by family and friends. ___ ___

Practical Facts and Suggestions about What to Do if Raped

1. Get to a safe place.
2. Call the police (911) and call a friend to be with you. The local rape crisis center has a 24-hour hot line and volunteers who will take you to the hospital and to the police if you wish.
3. Many people's first instinct is to take a shower and change. Although it is natural to want to "cleanse" oneself, *don't* wash, douche, change clothes, throw away clothes, or straighten up your apartment before going to the hospital or the police station. This is all evidence and needs to be preserved.
4. Arrange for transportation to and from a hospital or a physician. The police or the local rape crisis center can help you. If you prefer, you can arrange transportation with a friend.
5. *Go to a hospital or a private physician.* There are several important reasons that you should:

    a. Treatment for the prevention of *venereal disease.*
    b. Treatment for the prevention of *pregnancy.*
    c. A pelvic examination to check and treat *internal injuries.*
    d. Examination and treatment of *external injuries.*
    e. Gathering of *medical evidence* for possible legal prosecution.
    f. Counseling or referral for counseling for *emotional upset,* and for help in dealing with family, friends, and work, and with the police investigation and court.
    g. It is important to return for a follow-up medical appointment within six weeks for tests to make sure VD was effectively treated and for a pregnancy test if indicated.

6. The hospital does not routinely report the crime to the police. It is *your* choice and *your* responsibility to report the crime to the police.
7. You may want to stay with a friend. If you do, let the hospital and police know your temporary address.
8. If you decide not to go to the police, write down all the details of the assault and save them in case you change your mind. You should include a detailed description of your assailant, the time, the place, any conversation, his behavior, your behavior, sexual details, threats, etc. In estimating time, distance, or the assailant's build, give a range, for example, "I first saw him between 8:00 P.M. and 8:15 P.M. He was approximately 10–15 feet away. He was 5'10" and weighed around 185–200 pounds."
9. If you intend to follow the case to court, it is important to go immediately to a hospital or the police. Delays may be used in court later by the defense attorney to discredit your credibility.
10. *If you contact the police,* the following procedure will be followed:

    a. A responding unit arrives (usually a uniformed patrol officer).
    b. You will be asked to give a description of the assailant, and the patrol officer will arrange to collect material evidence; the officer is primarily concerned with your well-being and will take you to the hospital for an examination.

    c. A detective will be assigned to investigate the case. You should be aware that you may be asked more than once to go into detail concerning the rape. You may be asked to look through photographs to see if you can identify the assailant.

    d. If a suspect is apprehended, you will be asked to make an identification.

11. *If you decide to testify in court,* you should prepare yourself first by going over testimony with a friend or a counselor. Since the state brings the charges against the defendant, there is no need for you to hire a lawyer. The district attorney will represent your interests. You have the right to talk to the district attorney *before* your court appearance. The better prepared you are for court, the easier it will be for you. Familiarize yourself with what to expect: ask questions about procedures, privacy, whatever may be of concern to you.

12. The stages of legal prosecution are:

    a. *Probable cause hearing.* The first step at which the victim, the witnesses, and the defendant are present. You will be expected to testify, and you will be cross-examined by the defendant's lawyer. No jury is present; the case is heard by a judge, who decides whether the case should be referred to the grand jury.

    b. *Grand jury.* Just the victim appears before the grand jury, which is a closed hearing. The defendant is not present. No cross-examination occurs. The victim tells her story to the grand jury, which decides whether to indict the defendant. If an indictment is given, the case is referred to superior court.

    c. *Superior court.* The full trial with victim, defendant, and jury present occurs here. There is presentation of evidence and cross-examination. It is here that a verdict is reached and the defendant is sentenced.

The process can take as long as a year before the case comes to trial in the superior court. In certain instances, the general public may be excluded from either or both the probable cause hearing and the jury trial in superior court (the public is always excluded from the grand jury.) Ask your district attorney to explain the procedure to you.

13. Remember that it helps to talk to friends, family, or counselors because rape is a life crisis that can be disruptive for a time limited period. Like other crises, the rape crisis can stir up a lot of feelings and worries. It takes time to come to terms with such a major stress. This is *normal.* Women commonly experience some self-blame and guilt, anger, isolation, and helplessness as well as fear. Parents, spouses, boyfriends, and friends will all react to the rape. Sometimes their reactions can be worrisome to the victim. Counseling services are available for victims and their families.

[List resources available such as area hospitals with rape services, local rape crisis centers and hot lines, and victim–witness assistances programs provided by the court system.]

Safety Precautions to Avoid Assault

GENERAL PRECAUTIONS

Be aware that assaults, including rape, can happen to anyone, at any time, anywhere. Observe your environment and be alert.

Know your neighborhood and neighbors. Look for potential danger areas and safety areas. What stores, etc., are open late and may serve as shelters; who is likely to be home. Take note of unlighted or little-traveled areas and avoid them when possible.

Trust your gut feeling. If someone looks suspicious to you, get to a safe place and call the police. It is better to be embarrassed than to be hurt.

Be familiar with your own limitations and think about how you react under stress. Some women can respond effectively by physical struggle or fighting, others by flight and running, and others by distraction, screaming, or talking. What is your style?

Never hitchhike and don't accept rides from strangers.

Always carry enough money for an emergency phone call or taxi ride.

If you are assaulted and you see a weapon, your first priority is to not get hurt. Use your good judgment. Some of the tactics described may not be appropriate.

PRECAUTIONS AT HOME

Make your home as burglar-proof as possible. If it is a new residence, change the locks on all doors, and install locks on the windows and *use* them.

Always ask a repairman or a deliveryman for identification before opening the door. Check with their supervisor by phone if you are suspicious.

If someone wants to use your phone, offer to make the call for him rather than letting him into your house.

If a deliveryman has a package for a neighbor who is not home, ask him to leave it outside. Wait a sufficient length of time (30 minutes) to make sure he has left before you open the door.

Keep your curtains drawn at night to keep yourself from being observed and your home from being cased.

Do not reveal that you are home alone. If the doorbell rings, yell, "I'll get it, Joe" (or whatever male name you prefer).

Never list your first name on your mailbox or in the telephone directory; use initials.

Dogs are excellent protection. Even small ones can bark to sound an alarm.

If you are attacked in your apartment building, yell "Fire!" (It gets more response than screams or "Help!")

Report lewd or obscene phone calls. When you have such a call, hang up immediately or blow a loud police whistle into the mouthpiece.

It is better not to enter an elevator with a strange man or men if possible. Be sure the elevator has not been summoned to the roof or basement before getting on. Stand near the control panel so that you can push the alarm button if necessary.

Insist that your apartment manager keep hallways, entrances, and surrounding grounds well-lighted. Insist that there be a secure lock on apartment doors.

Don't release apartment lobby doors for people you do not know. If they are visiting someone in the building, *that* person will know them and let them in.

Carry your keys in your hand when entering your house or apartment. Don't fumble for them in your purse.

If someone drives you home, ask the person to wait until you are safely inside.

Precautions on the Street

Know where you are going and don't look lost. Get clear directions ahead of time and have the phone number of your destination.

Walk briskly and confidently and be alert to your surroundings.

Walk close to the curb, except when a car pulls up.

Choose well-lighted streets, and avoid streets where there are lots of bars.

Be familiar with your own frequently used routes.

If you are walking and you get the feeling that you are being followed, turn around and look. If anyone looks suspicious, cross the street and walk in the opposite direction.

If you are walking and being followed by a car, walk in the opposite direction the car is traveling and go to the nearest open store, neighbor, etc.

If you are approached or grabbed on the street, make a scene and try to run away. Scream, yell, or throw a rock or shoe through the nearest lighted window to attract attention.

Precautions in the Car

Keep cars doors locked at all times, including when you are riding in the car. Assailants have been known to jump into cars at stop lights.

Look into your back seat before you get into the car.

Always carry a road flare to signal when you have car trouble. *It* should be outside the car, not you.

If you have car trouble and have to pull over, keep your doors locked and your windows up. If no one is nearby, jump out and raise the hood and get back into the car and lock it. If someone stops and offers to help you, ask him to call the police or a garage. *Do not open your door.*

Do not stop to help a motorist. Think of your safety first, and be a "good Samaritan" by stopping at the nearest phone and calling for help.

Separate your house and your car keys when you leave your car for repairs. The garage man could make a duplicate of your house key.

Do not label your keys with your name or address.

Never pick up a hitchhiker.

If you believe that you are being followed by another car, don't pull into your driveway. Drive straight to the nearest police station or fire station and honk your horn. Do not leave your car until you are sure that it is safe.

PRECAUTIONS ON THE BUS OR SUBWAY

If you are waiting for the subway alone and the station is deserted, keep your back against a wall in a well-lighted section.

Stand near the change booth or near a group of people. Do not wander off by yourself.

While waiting for the bus, stand away from the curb until the bus arrives. If the bus is nearly empty, sit near the driver.

If you are bothered by a man on the bus or the subway, don't get off at your normal stop unless it is well lighted and well populated. Inform the driver of the trouble.

Index